NEW UNGUENT BASES AND LOTIONS

Formulae and Uses

By

ISAAC KENNETH HOFFMAN, B.S., PHARM.D.

Research Staff, U. C. L. A., School of Medicine, Division of Dermatology; Consulting Chemist

With Foreword by

THOMAS H. STERNBERG, M.D.

Professor of Dermatology
U. C. L. A. Medical Center

1957

CHEMICAL PUBLISHING CO., INC.

212 Fifth Avenue New York 10, N. Y.

New Unguent Lotions and Bases
Formulae and Uses

ISBN: 978-0-8206-0170-0

Chemical Publishing Company:
www.chemical-publishing.com
www.chemicalpublishing.net

First edition:

© **Chemical Publishing Company, Inc.** – New York, 1957
Second Impression:
Chemical Publishing Company, Inc. - 2013

Printed in the United States of America

FOREWORD

As a dermatologist, the work of Dr. Hoffman has held a special interest for me since much of dermatological therapy is based on administration of various medicaments to the skin. It is, therefore, of obvious importance that the physician should be well informed of the various lotions and unguent vehicles that are available and the properties they possess. Some of these are as follows: compatibility, consistency, release of active ingredients, absence of irritation, ease of removal, and finally esthetic value. It is equally obvious that for the physician alone to be aware of the attributes of an acceptable vehicle for topical medicaments is of little value if the individuals responsible for compounding do not prepare a satisfactory product. This applies to all the professions concerned whether they are in small or large commercial practice.

The original material presented in this volume is noteworthy because of the comprehensiveness with which the work is treated. For the first time, many types of excellent topical preparations have been made available to physicians, pharmacists, and chemists in a book written primarily for those in the dermatological and allied fields. As a ready reference, the advantages offered in the saving of time and effort is indeed commendable. The progress and improvement of vehicles for application to the skin, such as those included in this book, serve as a valuable link in the achievement of more satisfactory therapeutic response. It is also gratifying to observe that the preparations found on these pages are esthetically desirable for all forms of treatment.

The simplicity and scope of material in this book should be of benefit to those whose time and familiarity is, by necessity, limited. The author's wide experience contributes much toward a greater appreciation and understanding of good dermatological unguents and lotions.

THOMAS H. STERNBERG M.D.
Professor of Dermatology
University of California
Medical Center
Los Angeles, California

TO MY MOTHER AND FATHER

AUTHOR'S PREFACE

A reference and guide to the more advanced types of unguent bases and lotions has long been needed by the pharmaceutical, medical, and allied professions. The efforts of the author have been rewarded by the satisfaction gained in filling this need.

For the pharmacist, this book opens a wide field of reference and application to topical pharmaceutical preparations. From these formulae, he may choose those which are most satisfactory for his needs. He can utilize them as stock vehicles or use the diverse data as a source of information when advising the physician.

For the physician, this book will serve as a ready reference and formula guide to the various classes of dermatological products. Its value as a prescribing aid is enhanced by the description included with each formula. It has also the advantage that it lists specific preparations which can be used for special purposes.

For the pharmaceutical manufacturer, the formulae in this book can be of great value for commercial product development. The fine appearance, economy, safety, and ease of manufacture of the products listed, will make them especially suitable for pharmaceutical preparations.

For the cosmetic manufacturer, the versatility and special characteristics of the preparations described in the book present many interesting possibilities for commercial application. They can be combined with all types of perfumes, colors, or other cosmetic materials. As luxury products, these formulations are well chosen because of their attractiveness, effectiveness, safety, economy and ease of manufacture.

For use as a text, this book is of practical value, because it covers extensively the various classes of emulsified pharmaceutical preparations for topical use. Simple mixtures, solutions, or suspensions are not included. The descriptive material offers useful information to students of pharmacy, medicine, and related fields.

For the library, too, this book can be used as a reference, which covers most of the information available in this somewhat limited field. It is a good source for those whose diverse interests touch on this subject. As the lack of compiled material on unguent base and lotion emulsions is sorely evident, the author has taken great pains to put within easy reach the more advanced and practical formulae, methods of preparation, and uses.

In order to make the writing of a book, such as this, worth while, its need and utility must be established. This thought has been considered very carefully and the conclusions evolved are as follows: The information presented here is an application of theory to practice. All of the preparations described have been tried in the laboratory and have been found useful. They can be compounded with a minimum of expenditure in money, time, and effort. Only a few ingredients are necessary for all the classes of vehicles. The differences are created by varying the proportions of the same substances. Additional advantages of these unguent base and lotion formulae are the constant availability and proven safety of the individual ingredients.

The subject matter will satisfy a need for those who are constantly searching for better products. Large sums of money are expended by our drug and cosmetic manufacturing industry on research in order to obtain a desirable characteristic so that a preparation will be, for example, stainless or greaseless. The vehicles listed in this book are attractive, comfortable, versatile, and readily removable.

Every effort has been made to present the subject matter in a clear and concise manner. These new, practical formulae have been developed and tested by the author. This is the only book which is devoted solely to emulsified unguent bases and lotions.

ACKNOWLEDGEMENTS

The author wishes to express his appreciation to Dean Alva G. Hall and Professor Orville H. Miller of the University of Southern California, College of Pharmacy, as well as to Mr. Charles G. Towne, Chief Pharmacist of the Veterans Administration Hospital in West Los Angeles, California. Their kindness, advice, and cooperation have been an inspiration which will long be remembered.

My thanks are also due to Dr. Marion B. Sulzberger, Professor and Chairman, Department of Dermatology and Syphilology, New York University Postgraduate Medical School and to Dr. Thomas H. Sternberg, Professor of Medicine (Dermatology), the University of California, Los Angeles, School of Medicine for reading the manuscript and their valued suggestions.

CONTENTS

Foreword 3

Author's Preface 7

Acknowledgments 9

CHAPTER ONE

Introduction 11

CHAPTER TWO

Washable Oil-in-Water Unguent Bases 19

CHAPTER THREE

Washable Oil-in-Water Lotions 65

CHAPTER FOUR

Nonwashable Water-in-Oil Unguent Bases 108

CHAPTER FIVE

Nonwashable Water-in-Oil Lotions 120

CHAPTER SIX

Washable Anhydrous Oil-in-Water Unguent Bases 130

CHAPTER SEVEN

Nonwashable Anhydrous Water-in-Oil Unguent Bases 136

Bibliography 141

Index 146

Chapter One

INTRODUCTION

The unguent bases and lotions used in dermatological treatment can be quite greaseless, comfortable, and pleasing to the eye. The great advances in the field of emulsions have made possible the creation of stable, pleasant-feeling, nonirritable vehicles. Additional advantages are economy and facility of preparation. There are numerous other advantages, such as ease of removal, absorptive action, wide compatibility, etc., which will be discussed later in more detail.

The new unguent bases and lotions are white and creamlike. They create a sensation of coolness when applied to the skin. This is due to the slow evaporation of water from the emulsion. The evaporation, in turn, permits the escape of heat from the skin surface. The absorptive power of these bases permits the taking up of dermal excretory and secretory products. This property is especially valuable where irritable and purulent fluids are elaborated. The older, more greasy unguents and lotions had a tendency to cause congestion of the skin with subsequent irritation. This discomfort was produced by retarded drainage and restricted evaporation of these excretory products. Thus, the older vehicles encouraged heat retention which contributed to the discomfort.

The properties of a good unguent base or lotion are as follows:

Compatibility with most medicinal agents

Efficient release of therapeutic agents to the skin

Sufficient absorptive action to take up liquids

Nonirritability

Easy removal

Stability

Economy

Good appearance

The new unguent bases have a liquid content of approximately 50 percent. The lotions contain about 90 percent liquid. This consists primarily of water and/or oil. There may, at times, be a variation of this percentage. In the compounding of an unguent base or lotion, the water-soluble substances are dissolved in the aqueous phase and the oil-soluble ingredients are dissolved in the oil phase. The water-soluble and water-dispersible agents most generally used are presented in tables 1 and 2 which list also the common oil-soluble and oil-dispersible ingredients.

To compound a satisfactory unguent base or lotion, it is usually necessary to utilize substances that are both hydrophilic and lipophilic. The hydrophilic agents are associated with the aqueous phase and the lipophilic agents with the oil phase. The two groups, which are normally immiscible, are attracted to each other by surface-active, or emulsifying, agents.

Much credit must be given to colloid chemists for the progress and development of new, effective surface-active agents. Emulsifying agents facilitate the combination of immiscible substances by reducing their surface and interfacial tensions, thus making good, stable emulsions possible. To form emulsions, the ingredients must be reduced to a liquid state. If solids of low melting points are used, heat can readily liquefy them. Surface-active agents are both hydrophilic and lipophilic and thus are able to form a link between water-soluble and oil-soluble substances. The hydrophilic portion of the molecule may be a sulfonate, carboxylate or glycol group. The lipophilic portion may be a long carbon chain, such as a fatty acid group. For example, sodium sulfethyl oleate (a sodium alkyl sulfonate) consists of the following two portions:

$C_{17}H_{33}COO^-$	and	$CH_2CH_2SO_3Na^+$
Lipophilic		Hydrophilic

Surface-active agents are divided into three main classes, depending on the ionic charges they provide. They may be positively charged, negatively charged, or carry no charge at all. The positively charged surface-active agents are called cationic, those negatively charged are anionic and those without charge are nonionic. The ionic designation denotes the portion of the molecule which conveys the emulsifying properties. For example, the quaternary ammonium salts, such as benzalkonium chloride, are cationic. Soaps and sulfates of long-chain aliphatic alcohols, such as sodium lauryl sulfate, are anionic. Glyceryl esters of fatty acids and sorbitol compounds of fatty acids, such as glyceryl monostearate or sorbitan monooleate, are nonionic.

Surface-active agents produce emulsions of two types: oil-in-water or water-in-oil emulsions. A surface-active agent which exerts greater attraction on one phase than on the other determines the type of emulsion formed. For example, sodium lauryl sulfate is more soluble in the aqueous phase and, therefore, tends to form oil-in-water emulsions. In other words, the choice of the emulsifying agent for producing a specific type of emulsion depends to a great deal on the medium in which the agent is soluble.

The terms *oil-in-water* and *water-in-oil* have a definite meaning in emulsion formulation and their definitions will be given as follows: Oil-in-water signifies that the oil particles are dispersed in the water, so that the water is the external phase and the oil, the internal phase. If the emulsion is of the water-in-oil type, the particles or droplets of the water are dispersed in the oil. In this case, the oil is the external phase and the water, the internal phase. Expressing this another way, the medium in which the surface-active agent is soluble is called the external phase. The physical character of the external phase governs the physical and chemical behavior of the emulsion to a large extent. If water forms the external phase of the unguent base or lotion, the resulting emulsion is washable. The oil-in-water type emulsion can take up additional amounts of water if necessary. Some water-soluble drugs may be incorporated in this emulsion readily without the use of additional liquid. Oily therapeutic agents can also be incorporated due to their attraction to the lipophilic portion of the emulsifying agent. The surface-active agent also tends to reduce the surface tension of added liquids. If the emulsifying agent is cationic, there may be some difficulty when an anionic substance is introduced, resulting in nonuniformity or breaking of the emulsion. In this case, a nonionic surface active agent should be used. When large quantities of water-insoluble (oleaginous) substances are to be incorporated, emulsion bases and lotions of a lower aqueous content, or of the water-in-oil type, should be used.

Water-in-oil unguent bases and lotions are not readily washable. They produce a feeling of oiliness on the skin, but are able to absorb large quantities of aqueous or fatty matter. These emulsions are useful where a substantial proportion of oily emollient is desirable. If cholesterol is combined with this type of vehicle, increased dermal penetration is usually obtained. The water-in-oil emulsion vehicles are employed where more direct contact of oil with the skin is desirable or where washability is not wanted. They exert a greater protective action, but are less comfortable. As a vehicle, they are more efficient for carrying large amounts of oleaginous materials.

There are several ingredients in the new unguent bases and lotions which are suitable for both oil-in-water and water-in-oil emulsions. A good example is stearyl alcohol. This fatty acid derivative is normally oil soluble due to its long carbon chain. It also contains a hydroxyl group which tends to make it water soluble. Thus similar fatty alcohols, such as cetyl alcohol, are also hydrophilic even in water-in-oil emulsions.

Typical representatives of the nonionic emulsifiers are the sorbitol and glyceryl esters of fatty acids. Sorbitol, which is related to the sugars, is a partially dehydrated polyhydric alcohol. When used alone, in liquid form, it serves as a glycerin substitute because it, too, has emollient and humectant properties. Fatty acids, when combined with sorbitol, yield nonionic surface-active agents. Sorbitan oleate, stearate, or laurate forms water-in-oil emulsions because it is dispersible in oil. If a polyoxyethylene group is added to these compounds, their hydrophilic properties are enhanced making them water dispersible. This, in turn, permits the formation of oil-in-water emulsions. Here again the dual action of surface-active agents is illustrated. The three hydroxyl groups in the sorbitol portion and the polyoxyethylene groups supply the hydrophilic action. The fatty acid portion of the molecule is responsible for the lipophilic activity. A trade-marked name for oil-soluble sorbitol derivatives is Spans* and for water-soluble sorbitol derivatives, Tweens.*

Another interesting group of nonionic emulsifiers includes the polyethylene glycol derivatives, which are marketed as Carbowaxes.† Most of them have a molecular weight of more than 1000. They are stable, water soluble and nonvolatile. Their density is directly proportional to their molecular weight. Thus Carbowax 4000 is harder

*Atlas Powder Co., Wilmington, Del.
†Carbide & Carbon Chemicals Co., New York, N. Y.

than Carbowax 1500. Therefore, polyethylene glycols, which vary from liquids to hard waxy solids, are well suited for use in unguent bases and lotions. They can be employed as wax substitutes to improve consistency or can be used in anhydrous bases to lend viscosity and body. Being water soluble, they do not interfere with washability of the unguent base. It should be noted that bases containing polyethylene glycols tend to become less viscous when too much water is added. This is due to the solubility in water of these glycols.

The washable unguent bases and lotions, which are the oil-in-water types, have many advantages over most others. They are easily removed from the epidermal surfaces by application of water or by simple wiping. This is of importance where removal from painful or sloughing areas is necessary.

Most emulsion bases and lotions are subject to some mold growth, making the addition of inhibitors necessary. Propyl and methyl para-aminobenzoate, known as the parabens, are best suited for this purpose.

The water content of the new unguent bases and lotions is protected by proper closure of the containers. A well-balanced formula should contain sufficient glycerin or other similar agents, which act as humectants and thus retard water evaporation. Being hygroscopic, they tend to attract moisture, thus maintaining an equilibrium between water loss and water gain.

When the new unguent bases and lotions are used alone, they serve as simple emollients and protective agents. However, the prime function of these preparations is to act as a vehicle or carrier for therapeutic substances prescribed by the physician.

Oil-in-water emulsions generally provide the means for epidermic action only. The degree of penetration into the skin of an unguent base or lotion or of medicinal agents is primarily determined by the physician and not by the pharmacist or chemist. He is best qualified to include the most desirable agents for individual treatment.

Lanolin, which increases the dermal penetration of an unguent or lotion, has been omitted from the formulae in this volume. The physician may include it if he chooses.

The anhydrous bases are hydrophilic. Some are designed to be very absorptive, while others are made to be primarily nonaqueous. These bases may be washable or nonwashable. Those able to take up large amounts of water are called absorption bases. The washable types consist largely of polyethylene glycols and/or methyl cellulose mixtures. The nonwashable bases are composed mainly of petrolatum and a water-in-oil type of dispersing agent. These are absorptive and oilier than the washable bases.

Water-sensitive therapeutic agents, e.g., antibiotics, are reduced in potency or hydrolyzed in the presence of water. Therefore, anhydrous bases are used with these for effective therapy. The new anhydrous bases are also more pleasant to use than the older greasy, foul-smelling vehicles.

Homogenization, which reduces particle size and promotes dispersion, thus increasing emulsion stability, should be used whenever possible.

Unguent bases containing a very high percentage (over 50 percent) of water should not be used for water-insoluble drugs, such as salicylic acid, sulfur, and large amounts of oil. The formulae in this book were specially created to encompass as wide a range of application as possible.

TABLE 1

COMMON SURFACE-ACTIVE AGENTS

WATER SOLUBLE: PRODUCE O/W EMULSIONS

Type	*Example*	*Class*
Glyceryl Esters	Glyceryl Monostearate	Nonionic
Glycol Derivatives	Polyethylene Glycol Monostearate	Nonionic
Amine Derivatives	Triethanolamine	Nonionic
Polyoxyethylene Derivatives of Sorbitol Fatty Acid Esters	Tweens	Nonionic
Natural Gums	Acacia	Nonionic
Sulfated Fatty Acid Derivatives	Sodium Lauryl Sulfate	Anionic
Cellulose Derivatives	Methyl Cellulose	Nonionic
Soaps	Sodium Stearate	Anionic

OIL SOLUBLE: PRODUCE W/O EMULSIONS

Type	*Example*	*Class*
Lanolin Derivatives	Cholesterol and Oxycholesterol	Anionic
Sorbitol Fatty Acid Esters	Spans	Nonionic
Fatty Alcohols	Cetyl Alcohol	Nonionic
Metallic Salts	Sodium Borate (Borax)	Cationic

TABLE 2

COMMON INGREDIENTS OF UNGUENT BASES AND LOTIONS

Water Soluble		Oil Soluble	
Name	*Function*	*Name*	*Function*
Glycerin	Emollient Humectant Texture aid Spreading aid	Cetyl Alcohol	Plasticizer Texture aid Absorption aid Emulsion aid
Propylene Glycol	Emollient Humectant Texture aid Spreading aid	Stearyl Alcohol	Plasticizer Texture aid Absorption aid Emulsion aid
Sorbitol	Emollient Humectant	Stearic Acid	Plasticizer Texture aid Absorption aid Emulsion aid
Polyethylene Glycols	Plasticizer Wax substitute	Beeswax	Plasticizer Emulsion aid Texture aid
Methyl Cellulose	Plasticizer	Petrolatum	Plasticizer Emulsion aid Drug carrier Texture aid Emollient
Water	Emulsion aid Solvent Washability aid Bulk donor Drug carrier	Liquid Petrolatum	Emulsion aid Emollient Texture aid Drug carrier
Methyl Paraben (Methyl Parabenzoate)	Mold inhibitor	Spermaceti	Plasticizer Texture aid Emulsion aid Absorption aid
Propyl Paraben (Propyl Parabenzoate)	Mold inhibitor	Cholesterol	Absorption aid Penetration aid
Glyceryl Monostearate	Plasticizer Emulsion aid Texture aid	Lanolin	Absorption aid Plasticizer Penetration aid

For some time, there have been conflicting reports regarding the efficient release of medication from unguent bases. There have also been mixed findings regarding the causes of drug inactivation. Some surface-active agents and several unguent-base compounds are said to neutralize the therapeutic action of drugs. There is insufficient evidence to justify a definite stand in this matter. There is no doubt that in some specific instances, therapeutic, chemical, or physical incompatibility does occur in unguent bases and lotions, but much more investigation must be conducted before definite conclusions can be drawn. In the case of antibiotics, however, the author feels that specific unguent bases should be prescribed. Antibiotics are very complex and sensitive compounds. They vary greatly in physical and chemical characteristics and reactivity. The unguent bases and lotions which are to serve as vehicles for an antibiotic should be specially adapted to conform with its behavior. Thus the physical, chemical, and therapeutical characteristics of the drug can be preserved. Careful tests should be made for the examination of antibiotic unguents and lotions to determine the drug stability, compatibility, and release.

Chapter Two

WASHABLE OIL-IN-WATER UNGUENT BASES

BUFFABASE

		grams
A.	Stearic Acid	8.000
	Self-Emulsifying Glyceryl Monostearate	3.000
	White Petrolatum	17.000
	White Beeswax	6.000
	Liquid Petrolatum	3.000
B.	Sodium Lauryl Sulfate	1.000
	Glycerin	4.000
	Distilled Water	58.000
	Methyl Paraben	0.015
	Propyl Paraben	0.015

Heat *A* to 75 °C. Heat *B* to 75 °C. on a water bath. Add *B* to *A* slowly, stirring until congealed.

This is a smooth-textured base of medium body. It is compatible with the majority of dermatological agents. This vehicle is very satisfactory for use with semisolid and liquid medication, such as ichthammol, balsam of Peru, or boric acid solution. When employed alone, it is an effective emollient and protective agent which is very convenient for general-purpose work.

EXOBASE

		grams
A.	Cetyl Alcohol	12.000

Stearyl Alcohol	10.000
Liquid Petrolatum	13.000
White Beeswax	6.000
B. Sodium Lauryl Sulfate	1.000
Distilled Water	58.000
Methyl Paraben	0.015
Propyl Paraben	0.015

Heat *A* to 70°C. Heat *B* to 70° C. on a water bath. Add *B* to *A* slowly, stirring until congealed.

This gives a smooth, medium-bodied base which combines well with the majority of therapeutic agents. It does not absorb liquids well and is, therefore, more suitable for use with viscous or powdered medicaments. Balsam of Peru or ichthammol can be readily incorporated.

MODIBASE

	grams
A. Self-Emulsifying Glyceryl Monostearate	8.000
Stearic Acid	5.000
White Petrolatum	35.000
B. Distilled Water	52.000
Methyl Paraben	0.015
Propyl Paraben	0.015

Heat *A* to 75°C. Heat *B* to 75°C. on a water bath. Add *B* to *A* slowly, stirring until congealed.

This is a nonionic vehicle of smooth texture and heavy body. It is compatible with most therapeutic agents and absorbs liquids well. To remove, simply wash with water. It is a good base for solutions, e.g., Burow's solution.

SOFBASE

	grams
A. Cetyl Alcohol	7.000
White Petrolatum	16.000
White Beeswax	5.000

B.	Glycerin	3.000
	Sodium Lauryl Sulfate	1.000
	Distilled Water	68.000
	Methly Paraben	0.015
	Propyl Paraben	0.015

Heat *A* to 70 °C. Heat *B* to 70 °C. on a water bath. Add *B* to *A* slowly, stirring until congealed.

This yields a soft, light-bodied preparation which spreads easily in a thin layer. It is convenient for use on large areas. It is practically greaseless and combines well with powdered medication. If used alone, it is an excellent emollient and gives a good unguent with zinc oxide or calomel.

ATHERBASE

		grams
A.	Spermaceti	8.000
	Stearyl Alcohol	5.000
	White Beeswax	4.000
B.	Liquid Sorbitol	3.000
	Glycerin	5.000
	Sodium Lauryl Sulfate	1.000
	Distilled Water	74.000
	Methyl Paraben	0.015
	Propyl Paraben	0.015

Heat *A* to 70 °C. Heat *B* to 70 °C. on a water bath. Add *B* to *A* slowly, stirring until congealed.

An attractive, soft-bodied vehicle results, which is compatible with most types of medicinal agents. It is suitable for general-purpose work or can be employed alone as an emollient and protective agent. This preparation combines very well with powdered drugs, such as β-naphthol, boric acid, and bismuth subgallate.

DONABASE

	grams
Self-Emulsifying Glyceryl Monostearate	17.000
White Petrolatum	19.000

Distilled Water	64.000
Methly Paraben	0.015
Propyl Paraben	0.015

Heat all together to 70 °C. on a water bath. Stir slowly until congealed.

This attractive nonionic unguent base of medium body has excellent absorbent properties. It is compatible with almost all kinds of medication and is especially suitable for use with sulfur or tar.

TRANSIBASE

		grams
A.	Stearic Acid	13.000
	Glycerin	6.000
	White Petrolatum	11.000
B.	Propylene Glycol	2.000
	Sodium Lauryl Sulfate	1.000
	Distilled Water	67.000
	Methyl Paraben	0.015
	Propyl Paraben	0.015

Heat *A* to 75 °C. Heat *B* to 75 °C. on a water bath. Add *B* to *A* slowly, stirring until congealed.

This homogeneous medium-bodied base is suitable for combination with many therapeutic agents. It can also serve as a fine emollient and protective agent. It takes up powdered drugs, such as benzocaine, sulfathiazole, and boric acid.

TOROBASE

		grams
A.	Cetyl Alcohol	18.000
	White Beeswax	2.000
B.	Glycerin	9.000
	Sodium Lauryl Sulfate	1.000
	Distilled Water	70.000
	Methyl Paraben	0.015
	Propyl Paraben	0.015

Heat *A* to 70 °C. Heat *B* to 70 °C. on a water bath. Add *B* to *A* slowly, stirring until congealed.

This vehicle of smooth, heavy consistency has a firm adhesive body. It absorbs liquids readily and can be used with a large number of therapeutic agents. It is removed easily with water and is a good base for use with coal tar or pine tar.

PERLBASE

		grams
A.	Stearyl Alcohol	9.000
	Cetyl Alcohol	12.000
	White Petrolatum	28.000
B.	Propylene Glycol	8.000
	Sodium Lauryl Sulfate	1.000
	Distilled Water	42.000
	Methyl Paraben	0.015
	Propyl Paraben	0.015

Heat *A* to 70 °C. Heat *B* to 70 °C. on a water bath. Add *A* to *B* slowly, stirring until congealed.

This homogeneous, firm, heavy-bodied unguent base has good adhesive qualities. It is relatively nongreasy. Most dermatological agents can be incorporated and is well suited for use with liquids. Balsam of Peru combines very well with this vehicle.

SPAROBASE

		grams
A.	Cetyl Alcohol	13.000
	White Petrolatum	27.000
	White Beeswax	2.000
B.	Propylene Glycol	7.000
	Sodium Lauryl Sulfate	1.000
	Distilled Water	50.000
	Methyl Paraben	0.015
	Propyl Paraben	0.015

Heat *A* to 70 °C. Heat *B* to 70 °C. on a water bath. Add *B* to *A* slowly stirring until congealed.

This softer type of base spreads easily and is convenient for application to large areas. It takes up powdered, insoluble solids very well and other drugs can also be added. Zinc oxide added to this base yields an attractive product.

EMOLIBASE

	grams
Self-Emulsifying Glyceryl Monostearate	14.000
White Petrolatum	21.000
Glycerin	3.000
Distilled Water	62.000
Methyl Paraben	0.015
Propyl Paraben	0.015

Heat all together to 70 °C. on a water bath. Stir slowly until congealed.

This is a soft, light-bodied base of the nonionic type. It has an excellent appearance and is good for general-purpose use. Sulfathiazole or ichthammol are very well dispersed in this vehicle. Without medication, it can serve as a very good greaseless emollient.

BARIBASE

		grams
A.	Spermaceti	8.000
	Cetyl Alcohol	5.000
	Stearic Acid	7.000
B.	Glycerin	12.000
	Sodium Lauryl Sulfate	1.000
	Distilled Water	67.000
	Methyl Paraben	0.015
	Propyl Paraben	0.015

Heat *A* to 75 °C. Heat *B* to 75 °C. on a water bath. Add *B* to *A* slowly, stirring until congealed.

This homogeneous, medium-bodied vehicle has good liquid absorption. It is compatible with the majority of dermatological agents and is, therefore, suitable for general-purpose use. It spreads readily, is practically greaseless, and rinses off quickly with water. It is very easily combined with powdered and oleaginous medications, such as sulfathiazole, calomel, and oil of cade.

DYNABASE

		grams
A.	Stearyl Alcohol	9.000
	Cetyl Alcohol	8.000
	White Petrolatum	13.000
	White Beeswax	2.000
B.	Propylene Glycol	7.000
	Sodium Lauryl Sulfate	1.000
	Distilled Water	60.000
	Methyl Paraben	0.015
	Propyl Paraben	0.015

Heat *A* to 70 °C. Heat *B* to 70 °C. on a water bath. Add *B* to *A* slowly, stirring until congealed.

This unguent base is of medium consistency and has good adhesive and absorption properties. It is quite greaseless and is quickly removed with water. It is very useful with oily liquids and also for general-purpose work. It combines easily with benzyl benzoate.

RIMBASE

	grams
Self-Emulsifying Glyceryl Monostearate	16.000
Glycerin	12.000
Beeswax	2.000
Distilled Water	70.000
Methyl Paraben	0.015
Propyl Paraben	0.015

Heat all together to 70 °C. on a water bath. Stir slowly until congealed.

This nonionic, medium-bodied vehicle is practically greaseless. It spreads readily and is compatible with almost all dermatological agents, but powdered drugs are more efficiently incorporated. Sulfathiazole or bismuth subgallate combine very well with this base.

AUTOBASE

		grams
A.	Cetyl Alcohol	15.000
	White Petrolatum	26.000

White Beeswax	3.000
B. Glycerin	7.000
Sodium Lauryl Sulfate	1.000
Distilled Water	48.000
Methyl Paraben	0.015
Propyl Paraben	0.015

Heat *A* to 70 °C. Heat *B* to 70 °C. on a water bath. Add *B* to *A* slowly, stirring until congealed.

The resulting smooth, white unguent base of medium body spreads easily and rinses off readily with water. It is good for general-purpose use in combination with most medicaments and especially with sulfathiazole.

LOGABASE

	grams
A. Stearic Acid	12.000
Stearyl Alcohol	7.000
B. Propylene Glycol	14.000
Sodium Lauryl Sulfate	1.000
Distilled Water	66.000
Methyl Paraben	0.015
Propyl Paraben	0.015

Heat *A* to 75 °C. Heat *B* to 75 °C. on a water bath. Add *B* to *A* slowly, stirring until congealed.

This firm, medium-bodied preparation lends itself well to combination with the majority of dermatological agents. When used alone, it is an efficient emollient and protective agent. This base can be used with oily liquids or semisolid medicaments, such as olive oil or balsam of Peru. It is washable.

DIPLOBASE

	grams
A. Self-Emulsifying Glyceryl Monostearate	11.000
Cetyl Alcohol	5.000
White Petrolatum	10.000
White Beeswax	5.000
B. Glycerin	6.000

	Distilled Water	63.000
	Methyl Paraben	0.015
	Propyl Paraben	0.015

Heat *A* to 70 °C. Heat *B* to 70 °C. on a water bath. Add *B* to *A* slowly, stirring until congealed.

This smooth, nonionic base is of medium body and quite greaseless. It is compatible with most medicinal agents, being especially well adapted for use with salicylic acid.

BORNIBASE

		grams
A.	Stearyl Alcohol	12.000
	Liquid Petrolatum	8.000
	White Petrolatum	18.000
B.	Liquid Sorbitol	5.000
	Sodium Lauryl Sulfate	1.000
	Distilled Water	56.000
	Methyl Paraben	0.015
	Propyl Paraben	0.015

Heat *A* to 70 °C. Heat *B* to 70 °C. on a water bath. Add *B* to *A* slowly, stirring until congealed.

This yields a fine-textured base of soft body and pleasant appearance. It can be applied, spread, and washed off easily. It is suitable for use on large areas. Most dermatological substances can be effectively incorporated, especially powdered drugs, such as Vioform and tannic acid.

BEMABASE

		grams
A.	Cetyl Alcohol	20.000
	White Petrolatum	17.000
B.	Sodium Lauryl Sulfate	1.000
	Glycerin	7.000
	Distilled Water	55.000
	Methyl Paraben	0.015
	Propyl Paraben	0.015

Heat *A* to 70 °C. Heat *B* to 70 °C. on a water bath. Add *B* to *A* slowly, stirring until congealed.

This nongreasy preparation is smooth in texture and very attractive in appearance. It is of medium consistency and is especially useful with powdered drugs. It is also a good general-purpose base.

HETRIBASE

		grams
A.	Liquid Petrolatum	20.000
	Stearyl Alcohol	17.000
	White Beeswax	2.000
B.	Sodium Lauryl Sulfate	1.000
	Glycerin	7.000
	Distilled Water	53.000
	Methyl Paraben	0.015
	Propyl Paraben	0.015

Heat *A* to 70 °C. Heat *B* to 70 °C. on a water bath. Add *B* to *A* slowly, stirring until congealed.

A smooth soft-bodied vehicle results, which can be spread easily and removed quickly. It is especially convenient for application to large areas. It is highly compatible with most therapeutic agents and is thus suitable for general-purpose work. It takes up powdered drugs, such as urea, talc, or calomel easily.

HUMABASE

		grams
A.	Cetyl Alcohol	28.000
	White Petrolatum	30.000
	White Beeswax	0.500
B.	Glycerin	10.000
	Sodium Lauryl Sulfate	1.000
	Distilled Water	30.500
	Methyl Paraben	0.015
	Propyl Paraben	0.015

Heat *A* to 75 °C. Heat *B* to 75 °C. on a water bath. Add *A* to *B* slowly, stirring until congealed.

This is a homogeneous base of firm consistency. It is liquid absorbent and adheres well. It is compatible with most types of medications and can be washed off easily with water. It is a convenient base for use with Burow's solution and boric acid solution.

BETABASE

		grams
A.	Stearic Acid	8.000
	Cetyl Alcohol	9.000
	White Petrolatum	20.000
	White Beeswax	2.000
B.	Propylene Glycol	5.000
	Sodium Lauryl Sulfate	1.000
	Distilled Water	55.000
	Methyl Paraben	0.015
	Propyl Paraben	0.015

Heat *A* to 75 °C. Heat *B* to 75 °C. on a water bath. Add *B* to *A* slowly, stirring until congealed.

A smooth, heavy bodied preparation of good adhesive and absorbent properties. It can be used as a simple emollient and protective agent or as a vehicle for therapeutic agents. It washes off quickly with warm water. Salicylic acid can be readily incorporated, resulting in a fine-textured preparation.

NOTOBASE

		grams
A.	Stearyl Alcohol	13.000
	White Petrolatum	28.000
	White Beeswax	1.000
B.	Propylene Glycol	7.000
	Sodium Lauryl Sulfate	1.000
	Distilled Water	50.000
	Methyl Paraben	0.015
	Propyl Paraben	0.015

Heat *A* to 70 °C. Heat *B* to 70 °C. on a water bath. Add *B* to *A* slowly, stirring until congealed.

This is a very firm and adhesive unguent base of heavy body which absorbs liquids readily and can be removed by washing with water. It is good for use with oily agents, such as olive and linseed oil, and crude coal tar.

HYLOBASE

		grams
A.	White Petrolatum	19.000
	Liquid Petrolatum	9.000
	Stearic Acid	9.000
	White Beeswax	1.000
B.	Propylene Glycol	4.000
	Sodium Lauryl Sulfate	1.000
	Distilled Water	57.000
	Propyl Paraben	0.015
	Methyl Paraben	0.015

Heat *A* to 75°C. Heat *B* to 75°C. on a water bath. Add *B* to *A* slowly, stirring until congealed.

This attractive, medium-bodied preparation is an excellent lubricant and protective agent. It can be combined with liquid or powdered medication, particularly phenol, camphor, urea, or castor oil. It is washable.

PERMIBASE

		grams
A.	Stearic Acid	15.000
	Polyethylene Glycol-1500*	15.000
B.	Glycerin	12.000
	Sodium Lauryl Sulfate	1.000
	Distilled Water	57.000
	Methyl Paraben	0.015
	Propyl Paraben	0.015

Heat *A* to 75°C. Heat *B* to 75°C. on a water bath. Add *B* to *A* slowly, stirring until congealed.

This firm heavy-bodied preparation spreads and adheres well. It can be removed quickly by rinsing with water. As a vehicle, it is highly compatible with all classes of medication. It is best adapted for use with oily liquids and semisolids, such as castor oil or crude coal tar.

---

*Carbide & Carbon Chemicals Co.

ROMABASE

	grams
Self-Emulsifying Glyceryl Monostearate	17.000
White Petrolatum	16.000
Glycerin	8.000
Distilled Water	59.000
Methyl Paraben	0.015
Propyl Paraben	0.015

Heat all together to 70°C. on a water bath. Stir slowly until congealed.

This is a smooth nonionic vehicle of medium body. It has good adhesive properties and excellent liquid absorption. It spreads readily and is easily removed with water. It may be used with all types of drugs.

BRIABASE

		grams
A.	Cetyl Alcohol	13.000
	White Petrolatum	5.000
	White Beeswax	2.000
B.	Glycerin	8.000
	Sodium Lauryl Sulfate	1.000
	Distilled Water	71.000
	Methyl Paraben	0.015
	Propyl Paraben	0.015

Heat *A* to 70°C. Heat *B* to 70°C. on a water bath. Add *B* to *A* slowly, stirring until congealed.

This firm, heavy-bodied base has excellent adhesive properties. It is suitable for general-purpose use alone or in combination. It absorbs liquids well and is particularly suited for use with salicylic acid.

RETROBASE

	grams
Polyethylene Glycol-1500*	12.000
Methyl Cellulose-1500†	8.000
Glycerin	10.000
Distilled Water	70.000
Methyl Paraben	0.015
Propyl Paraben	0.015

Heat all together to 75°C. on a water bath. Stir slowly until cool and smooth.

This yields a firm, medium-bodied, nonionic base of good texture and adherence. It has effective liquid absorption and spreading properties and is compatible with most medicinal agents. It can be rinsed off with water. Very satisfactory results are obtained when powdered drugs are added, such as resorcin or benzoic acid.

*Carbide & Carbon Chemicals Co.
†Dow Chemical Co.

OSLERBASE

		grams
A.	Stearic Acid	16.000
	Stearyl Alcohol	4.000
	White Petrolatum	9.000
	White Beeswax	5.000
B.	Propylene Glycol	5.000
	Sodium Lauryl Sulfate	1.000
	Distilled Water	60.000
	Methyl Paraben	0.015
	Propyl Paraben	0.015

Heat *A* to 75°C. Heat *B* to 75°C. on a water bath. Add *B* to *A* slowly, stirring until congealed.

This smooth-spreading, medium-bodied vehicle is well adapted for use with liquids or as a simple protective agent. Medications, such as camphor and menthol combinations, can be incorporated.

LARGOBASE

	grams
Spermaceti	7.000
Self-Emulsifying Glyceryl Monostearate	5.000
Methyl Cellulose 1500*	3.000
Glycerin	7.000
Distilled Water	78.000
Methyl Paraben	0.015
Propyl Paraben	0.015

Heat all together to 70 °C. on a water bath. Stir slowly until cool and smooth.

A well-balanced vehicle of medium body and fine texture results. It spreads easily, adheres well, and rinses off quickly with water. This nonionic base can be combined with all medicinal agents. It is very effective for general-purpose use or as an emollient and protective agent. It can be used with oily liquids and powdered drugs, such as pyrogallol or salicylic acid.

*Dow Chemical Co.

RENOBASE

		grams
A.	Cetyl Alcohol	9.000
	Stearyl Alcohol	5.000
	White Beeswax	2.000
	White Petrolatum	23.000
B.	Sodium Lauryl Sulfate	1.000
	Glycerin	5.000
	Distilled Water	55.000
	Methyl Paraben	0.015
	Propyl Paraben	0.015

Heat *A* to 70 °C. Heat *B* to 70 °C. on a water bath. Add *B* to *A* slowly, stirring until congealed.

This gives a fine-textured base of medium body. Without medication, it is a good greaseless emollient. It is suitable for general-purpose use, absorbs liquids, and takes up ammoniated mercury.

EVERBASE

		grams
A.	Self-Emulsifying Glyceryl Monostearate	15.000
	Cetyl Alcohol	5.000
	White Petrolatum	15.000
	White Beeswax	3.000
B.	Glycerin	5.000
	Distilled Water	57.000
	Methyl Paraben	0.015
	Propyl Paraben	0.015

Heat *A* to 70 °C. Heat *B* to 70 °C. on a water bath. Add *B* to *A* slowly, stirring until congealed.

This is a nonionic vehicle of medium consistency. It has good adhesive and absorption character with ready washability. It can be applied evenly and is quite greaseless. It is a convenient general-purpose base which is compatible with a great number of dermatological agents. It produces an excellent unguent with solutions of coal tar or ichthammol.

SUPRABASE

		grams
A.	Cetyl Alcohol	5.000
	Self-Emulsifying Glyceryl Monostearate	9.000
	White Petrolatum	5.000
	Liquid Petrolatum	15.000
	White Beeswax	5.000
B.	Glycerin	6,000
	Distilled Water	55.000
	Methyl Paraben	0.015
	Propyl Paraben	0.015

Heat *A* to 70 °C. Heat *B* to 70 °C. on a water bath. Add *B* to *A* slowly, stirring until congealed.

This yields a firm heavy-bodied preparation of good adhesive properties. It spreads easily and can be removed quickly with water. It absorbs liquids well and combines with ichthyol to an attractive, greaseless unguent.

DEBUBASE

		grams
A.	Stearic Acid	12.000
	Stearyl Alcohol	4.000
	White Petrolatum	20.000
	Liquid Petrolatum	10.000
	White Beeswax	4.000
B.	Sodium Lauryl Sulfate	1.000
	Distilled Water	49.000
	Methyl Paraben	0.015
	Propyl Paraben	0.015

Heat *A* to 75°C. Heat *B* to 75°C. on a water bath. Add *B* to *A* slowly, stirring until congealed.

A firm, heavy-bodied unguent base results which is suitable for use with aqueous or oily liquids, and rinses off easily with water. Phenol or methyl salicylate combines well with this base.

H BASE

		grams
A.	Cetyl Alcohol	7.000
	Stearyl Alcohol	3.000
	White Beeswax	4.000
	White Petrolatum	27.000
B.	Glycerin	8.000
	Sodium Lauryl Sulfate	1.000
	Distilled Water	50.000
	Methyl Paraben	0.015
	Propyl Paraben	0.015

Heat *A* to 70°C. Heat *B* to 70°C. on a water bath. Add *B* to *A* slowly, stirring until congealed.

This fine, medium-bodied base is suitable for general-purpose use. It is compatible with most dermatological agents or, if employed alone, is a good emollient and protective agent. It spreads smoothly and can be removed quickly with water. Cod liver oil or zinc oxide form a good unguent with this base.

DERABASE

		grams
A.	White Petrolatum	10.000
	Cetyl Alcohol	3.000
B.	Methyl Cellulose 1500*	3.000
	Glycerin	5.000
	Sodium Lauryl Sulfate	1.000
	Distilled Water	78.000
	Methyl Paraben	0.015
	Propyl Paraben	0.015

Heat *A* to 70°C. Heat *B* to 70°C. on a water bath. Add *B* to *A* slowly, stirring until cool and smooth.

This soft, smooth vehicle is suitable for general-purpose use because of its wide range of compatibility. It can be applied easily and is quickly removed with water. It is a good greaseless emollient. It takes up powdered drugs, such as ammoniated mercury or magnesium oxide.

*Dow Chemical Co.

SINTRABASE

		grams
A.	Spermaceti	18.000
	White Petrolatum	22.000
	White Beeswax	2.000
B.	Glycerin	6.000
	Sodium Lauryl Sulfate	1.000
	Distilled Water	51.000
	Methyl Paraben	0.015
	Propyl Paraben	0.015

Heat *A* to 70°C. Heat *B* to 70°C. on a water bath. Add *B* to *A* slowly, stirring until congealed.

This yields a soft, light-bodied base, which can serve as a good emollient. As a general-purpose vehicle, it spreads easily and can be used on large areas. Oil of cade and creosote combine well with this preparation.

ORNABASE

	grams
A. Cetyl Alcohol	4.000
Self-Emulsifying Glyceryl Monostearate	9.000
White Beeswax	2.000
White Petrolatum	38.000
B. Glycerin	4.00
Distilled Water	43.000
Methyl Paraben	0.015
Propyl Paraben	0.015

Heat *A* to 70°C. Heat *B* to 70°C. on a water bath. Add *B* to *A* slowly, stirring until congealed.

This firm, nonionic, heavy-bodied base has good adhesive and absorbent character. It can be employed with a great variety of therapeutic agents, such as lanolin and crude coal tar.

GRANBASE

	grams
A. Self-Emulsifying Glyceryl Monostearate	16.000
Stearyl Alcohol	7.000
White Beeswax	2.000
White Petrolatum	6.000
B. Glycerin	4.000
Distilled Water	65.000
Methyl Paraben	0.015
Propyl Paraben	0.015

Heat *A* to 70°C. Heat *B* to 70°C. on a water bath. Add *B* to *A* slowly, stirring until congealed.

This is a nonionic, firm, heavy-bodied base of good adhesive and absorption properties. It is compatible with practically all medicinal agents and is especially convenient for use with aqueous, oily, and alcoholic liquids. Crude coal tar or phenol combine readily with this vehicle.

PARMABASE

	grams
A. Stearic Acid	5.000

	Cetyl Alcohol	6.000
	White Beeswax	3.000
	White Petrolatum	28.000
B.	Glycerin	8.000
	Sodium Lauryl Sulfate	1.000
	Distilled Water	49.000
	Methyl Paraben	0.015
	Propyl Paraben	0.015

Heat *A* to 75°C. Heat *B* to 75°C. on a water bath. Add *B* to *A* slowly, stirring until congealed.

This is a medium-bodied unguent base of fine texture, smooth spreading, and good adhesive character. It is suited for general-purpose work or as a simple emollient and protective agent. Mixed with precipitated sulfur, it gives a good unguent.

ZONABASE

		grams
A.	Self-Emulsifying Glyceryl Monostearate	15.000
	White Petrolatum	42.000
B.	Glycerin	4.000
	Distilled Water	39.000
	Methyl Paraben	0.015
	Propyl Paraben	0.015

Heat *A* to 70°C. Heat *B* to 70°C. on a water bath. Add *B* to *A* slowly, stirring until congealed.

This nonionic unguent base has good compatibility with practically all therapeutic agents. It has heavier than average body and good adhesive and absorption properties. It is relatively greaseless and easily removable with water. It can be used with salicylic and benzoic acid.

LIBRABASE

		grams
A.	Stearyl Alcohol	13.000
	White Petrolatum	10.000
	White Beeswax	2.000

B.	Propylene Glycol	5.000
	Sodium Lauryl Sulfate	1.000
	Distilled Water	69.000
	Methyl Paraben	0.015
	Propyl Paraben	0.015

Heat *A* to 70°C. Heat *B* to 70°C. on a water bath. Add *A* to *B* slowly, stirring until congealed.

This yields a smooth, white lotion of medium body which spreads easily. It is a good preparation for general-purpose work in combination with most types of therapeutic agents. With a view to its good liquid absorption, it is a fine vehicle for lime water and camphor water.

ELMBASE

		grams
A.	Self-Emulsifying Glyceryl Monostearate	10.000
	White Beeswax	4.000
	White Petrolatum	20.000
	Stearyl Alcohol	4.000
B.	Glycerin	2.000
	Distilled Water	60.000
	Methyl Paraben	0.015
	Propyl Paraben	0.015

Heat *A* to 70°C. Heat *B* to 70°C. on a water bath. Add *B* to *A* slowly, stirring until congealed.

This is a smooth, nonionic vehicle of medium body. It is compatible with a great majority of dermatological agents and has good liquid-absorbent character. It removes easily with water. It is suitable for general-purpose work and takes up camphor and menthol well.

ARMABASE

		grams
A.	Cetyl Alcohol	13.000
	White Beeswax	3.000
B.	Glycerin	7.000
	Sodium Lauryl Sulfate	1.000
	Distilled Water	76.000

	Methyl Paraben	0.015
	Propyl Paraben	0.015

Heat *A* to 70°C. Heat *B* to 70°C. on a water bath. Add *B* to *A* slowly, stirring until congealed.

A smooth vehicle of medium body results, which spreads easily and can be removed quickly with water. It is practically greaseless and thus enhances comfort. This base is well adapted for use with powdered drugs, such as talc, starch, or boric acid.

PREGOBASE

		grams
A.	Self-Emulsifying Glyceryl Monostearate	11.000
	Stearyl Alcohol	19.000
	Liquid Petrolatum	6.000
B.	Polyethylene Glycol—1500*	16.000
	Glycerin	16.000
	Sodium Lauryl Sulfate	1.000
	Distilled Water	31.000
	Methyl Paraben	0.015
	Propyl Paraben	0.015

Heat *A* to 75°C. Heat *B* to 75°C. on a water bath. Add *B* to *A* slowly, stirring until congealed.

This good, heavy-bodied base can absorb all types of liquid, as well as solid, medication. It is compatible with most classes of therapeutic agents and is, therefore, convenient for general-purpose work. It may be used with both aqueous solutions and oily liquids, such as rose water, benzyl benzoate, or olive oil.

*Carbide & Carbon Chemicals Co.

VARIBASE

		grams
A.	Stearic Acid	16.000
	White Beeswax	3.000
	Span-60*	8.000
B.	Tween-60*	8.000
	Distilled Water	65.000

Methyl Paraben	0.015
Propyl Paraben	0.015

Heat *A* to 85°C. Heat *B* to 85°C. on a water bath. Add *B* to *A* slowly, stirring until congealed.

This is a greaseless, nonionic vehicle having a soft, light body. It can combine with all types of medication, but is best suited for use with powdered drugs, such as resorcin or sulfathiazole.

*Atlas Powder Co.

LAURABASE

		grams
A.	Spermaceti	14.000
	Cetyl Alcohol	12.000
	White Petrolatum	18.000
B.	Sodium Lauryl Sulfate	1.000
	Distilled Water	55.000
	Methyl Paraben	0.015
	Propyl Paraben	0.015

Heat *A* to 70°C. Heat *B* to 70°C. on a water bath. Add *B* to *A* slowly, stirring until congealed.

This is a firm, heavy-bodied preparation of high viscosity and great adhesive power. It absorbs all types of liquids. Balsam of Peru is especially well accepted by this base.

KEBRABASE

		grams
A.	White Petrolatum	16.000
	Liquid Petrolatum	9.000
	White Beeswax	6.000
B.	Sodium Lauryl Sulfate	1.000
	Distilled Water	68.000
	Methyl Paraben	0.015
	Propyl Paraben	0.015

Heat *A* to 70°C. Heat *B* to 70°C. on a water bath. Add *B* to *A* slowly, stirring until congealed.

This smooth, soft-bodied vehicle can be used with most dermatological agents in liquid or powdered form. It will absorb semisolid and solid medication, such as crude coal tar, calamine, or ammoniated mercury. It is easily removed by rinsing with water.

CREMBASE

		grams
A.	Stearic Acid	12.000
	Self-Emulsifying Glyceryl Monostearate	5.000
	Liquid Petrolatum	19.000
B.	Glycerin	3.000
	Sodium Lauryl Sulfate	1.000
	Distilled Water	60.000
	Methyl Paraben	0.015
	Propyl Paraben	0.015

Heat *A* to 75°C. Heat *B* to 75°C. on a water bath. Add *B* to *A* slowly, stirring until congealed.

This gives a soft greaseless base of light body. It is compatible with the majority of therapeutic agents and is well suited for application to large areas. It spreads thinly and can be removed easily with water. Powdered or oily medication is best for combination with this vehicle. Starch or thymol iodide can be easily incorporated.

EQUABASE

		grams
A.	Stearyl Alcohol	5.000
	Spermaceti	8.000
	Self-Emulsifying Glyceryl Monostearate	5.000
	White Petrolatum	22.000
	Span-40*	8.000
B.	Tween-40*	4.000
	Distilled Water	48.000
	Methyl Paraben	0.015
	Propyl Paraben	0.015

Heat *A* to 80°C. Heat *B* to 80°C. on a water bath. Add *B* to *A* slowly, stirring until congealed.

This nonionic, heavy-bodied base has very good liquid absorbent properties. It is compatible with practically all therapeutic agents.

Precipitated sulfur or salicylic acid can be incorporated easily to form a smooth unguent. Tincture of benzoin can also be used.

---

*Atlas Powder Co.

PETTIBASE

		grams
A.	Cetyl Alcohol	14.000
	Stearyl Alcohol	4.000
	White Petrolatum	28.000
	White Beeswax	6.000
B.	Sodium Lauryl Sulfate	1.000
	Liquid Sorbitol	6.000
	Distilled Water	41.000
	Methyl Paraben	0.015
	Propyl Paraben	0.015

Heat *A* to 70°C. Heat *B* to 70°C. on a water bath. Add *B* to *A* slowly, stirring until congealed.

This heavy-bodied vehicle has good absorbency and adhesiveness. It can be easily spread on large areas without discomfort. Most drugs are compatible with this base. Liquids as well as powders, such as sulfur, may be incorporated.

KEYBASE

		grams
A.	Stearyl Alcohol	8.000
	Self-Emulsifying Glyceryl Monostearate	15.000
	White Petrolatum	12.000
	Liquid Petrolatum	8.000
B.	Glycerin	7.000
	Distilled Water	50.000
	Methyl Paraben	0.015
	Propyl Paraben	0.015

Heat *A* to 70°C. Heat *B* to 70°C. on a water bath. Add *B* to *A* slowly, stirring until congealed.

This is a medium-bodied nonionic, smooth-textured, and smooth-spreading base. It has excellent liquid absorbent properties and is quite greaseless. Most medicaments are compatible, making it suitable for general-purpose use. Methyl salicylate and camphor combine very well with this vehicle.

ALTABASE

		grams
A.	Spermaceti	5.000
	Stearyl Alcohol	20.000
	White Petrolatum	29.000
B.	Glycerin	10.000
	Sodium Lauryl Sulfate	1.000
	Distilled Water	35.000
	Methyl Paraben	0.015
	Propyl Paraben	0.015

Heat *A* to 70°C. Heat *B* to 70°C. on a water bath. Add *B* to *A* slowly, stirring until congealed.

This gives a firm, smooth-textured vehicle of heavy body with good adhesive character. It is quite greaseless and absorbent. Hydrous, oleaginous, and alcoholic liquids are compatible with this preparation. It is a good base for cod liver oil.

ETHIBASE

		grams
A.	Glyceryl Monostearate	20.000
	White Petrolatum	23.000
B.	Propylene Glycol	11.000
	Sodium Lauryl Sulfate	1.000
	Distilled Water	45.000
	Methyl Paraben	0.015
	Propyl Paraben	0.015

Heat *A* to 75°C. Heat *B* to 75°C. on a water bath. Add *B* to *A* slowly, stirring until congealed.

This is a very absorbent, medium-bodied preparation. It can be combined with a large number of drugs and is, therefore, useful for general-purpose work, especially for liquids. Salicylic acid and benzoic acid are easy to incorporate.

HASTIBASE

		grams
A.	Cetyl Alcohol	15.000
	Stearic Acid	3.000
	Liquid Petrolatum	10.000
B.	Polyethylene Glycol—1500*	26.000
	Glycerin	8,000
	Sodium Lauryl Sulfate	1.000
	Distilled Water	37.000
	Methyl Paraben	0.015
	Propyl Paraben	0.015

Heat *A* to 75°C. Heat *B* to 75°C. on a water bath. Add *B* to *A* slowly, stirring until congealed.

This firm, heavy-bodied vehicle has good liquid absorption. It can be incorporated with the majority of dermatological agents and is, therefore, well suited for general-purpose work, especially for alcoholic and nonaqueous liquids, such as a solution of coal tar or methyl salicylate. It is easily washed off with water.

*Carbide & Carbon Chemicals Co.

AMIBASE

		grams
A.	Stearyl Alcohol	19.000
	White Petrolatum	19.000
	White Beeswax	2.000
B.	Glycerin	6.000
	Sodium Lauryl Sulfate	1.000
	Distilled Water	53.000
	Methyl Paraben	0.015
	Propyl Paraben	0.015

Heat *A* to 70°C. Heat *B* to 70°C. on a water bath. Add *B* to *A* slowly, stirring until congealed

This adhesive, heavy-bodied vehicle is very useful for liquid absorption. It is relatively greaseless and compatible with many therapeutic agents. Solutions of sodium thiosulfate or olive oil combine very well with this base.

HELIBASE

		grams
A.	Cetyl Alcohol	10.000
	Stearyl Alcohol	10.000
	Self-Emulsifying Glyceryl Monostearate	8.000
	White Petrolatum	30.000
B.	Glycerin	6.000
	Sodium Lauryl Sulfate	1.000
	Distilled Water	35.000
	Methyl Paraben	0.015
	Propyl Paraben	0.015

Heat *A* to 75°C. Heat *B* to 75°C. on a water bath. Add *B* to *A* slowly, stirring until congealed.

This is a smooth, heavy-bodied base for general-purpose work. It spreads easily and can be removed readily with water. It is compatible with a wide range of therapeutic agents and absorbs liquids. Ammoniated mercury produces an excellent preparation with this base.

JEFBASE

		grams
A.	Spermaceti	15.000
	Cetyl Alcohol	7.000
	Stearyl Alcohol	3.000
	White Petrolatum	17.000
	Liquid Petrolatum	9.000
B.	Sodium Lauryl Sulfate	1.000
	Distilled Water	48.000
	Methyl Paraben	0.015
	Propyl Paraben	0.015

Heat *A* to 70°C. Heat *B* to 70°C. on a water bath. Add *B* to *A* slowly, stirring until congealed.

This is a good, general-purpose, nongreasy base of medium consistency. It is smooth and can be applied in an even layer. Powdered medication, such as zinc oxide or ammoniated mercury, can be incorporated well.

NYBASE

	grams
A. Stearic Acid	5.000
Self-Emulsifying Glyceryl Monostearate	6.000
Cetyl Alcohol	4.000
White Beeswax	1.000
White Petrolatum	30.000
B. Glycerin	8.000
Sodium Lauryl Sulfate	1.000
Distilled Water	45.000
Methyl Paraben	0.015
Propyl Paraben	0.015

Heat *A* to 75°C. Heat *B* to 75°C. on a water bath. Add *B* to *A* slowly, stirring until congealed.

This good, medium-bodied vehicle can be easily applied or removed. Powdered or liquid medicinal agents can be readily incorporated. Oil of cade and castor oil combine well with this base.

ALTIBASE

	grams
A. Self-Emulsifying Glyceryl Monostearate	5.000
Cetyl Alcohol	5.000
Stearyl Alcohol	5.000
White Beeswax	2.000
White Petrolatum	29.000
B. Glycerin	5.000
Sodium Lauryl Sulfate	1.000
Distilled Water	48.000
Methyl Paraben	0.015
Propyl Paraben	0.015

Heat *A* to 70°C. Heat *B* to 70°C. on a water bath. Add *B* to *A* slowly, stirring until congealed.

This is a smooth, medium-bodied preparation of good adhesive and absorption character. It can be employed with most types of medication and is especially useful with oily liquids, such as olive oil.

SEEBASE

		grams
A.	Cetyl Alcohol	10.000
	Stearyl Alcohol	5.000
	White Petrolatum	33.000
	White Beeswax	4.000
B.	Glycerin	9.000
	Sodium Lauryl Sulfate	1.000
	Distilled Water	38.000
	Methyl Paraben	0.015
	Propyl Paraben	0.015

Heat *A* to 70°C. Heat *B* to 70°C. on a water bath. Add *B* to *A* slowly, stirring until congealed.

This firm, adhesive, heavy-bodied vehicle has good liquid absorption. Most therapeutic agents are compatible with it. It combines well with oily and aqueous liquids. Vitamin A concentrate and camphor water are very easily incorporated.

BEVABASE

		grams
A.	Stearyl Alcohol	15.000
	White Beeswax	2.000
	Span-60*	7.000
B.	Tween-60*	4.000
	Distilled Water	72.000
	Methyl Paraben	0.015
	Propyl Paraben	0.015

Heat *A* to 85°C. Heat *B* to 85°C. on a water bath. Add *B* to *A* slowly, stirring until congealed.

This soft-bodied unguent base spreads easily in a thin layer and is practically greaseless. It is of the nonionic type and, therefore, compatible with a very large number of medicinal substances. It rinses off easily with water. It is well suited for use with powdered drugs. Sulfathiazole and chrysarobin combine very well with it.

---

*Atlas Powder Co.

ALPABASE

		grams
A.	Stearic Acid	17.000
	Cetyl Alcohol	5.000
B.	Sodium Lauryl Sulfate	1.000
	Glycerin	7.000
	Distilled Water	70.000
	Methyl Paraben	0.015
	Propyl Paraben	0.015

Heat *A* to 75°C. Heat *B* to 75°C. on a water bath. Add *B* to *A* slowly, stirring until congealed.

This soft, light-bodied vehicle is of smooth texture and spreads easily over large areas. It may be used as a simple protective or combined with powdered drugs, such as boric acid powder and starch.

STEFBASE

		grams
A.	Cetyl Alcohol	11.000
	White Petrolatum	30.000
	White Beeswax	4.000
B.	Glycerin	6.000
	Sodium Lauryl Sulfate	1.000
	Distilled Water	48.000
	Methyl Paraben	0.015
	Propyl Paraben	0.015

Heat *A* to 75°C. Heat *B* to 75°C. on a water bath. Add *B* to *A* slowly, stirring until congealed.

A smooth, medium-bodied vehicle of good adhesive character results. It is suitable for general-purpose work or as an emollient and can be washed off with water. Balsam of Peru and oil of cade are easy to incorporate.

SUNBASE

	grams
Self-Emulsifying Glyceryl Monostearate	17.000
White Petrolatum	33.000

Distilled Water	50.000
Methyl Paraben	0.015
Propyl Paraben	0.015

Heat all together to 65°C. on a water bath. Stir slowly until congealed.

This firm, nonionic, heavy-bodied vehicle has good adhesive character and is compatible with a large number of medicinal preparations, especially oily substances. Ichthammol and castor oil form very satisfactory unguents with this base.

STERABASE

	grams
A. Stearyl Alcohol	9.000
Cetyl Alcohol	4.000
White Petrolatum	23.000
Liquid Petrolatum	9.000
B. Sodium Lauryl Sulfate	1.000
Distilled Water	55.000
Methyl Paraben	0.015
Propyl Paraben	0.015

Heat *A* to 70°C. Heat *B* to 70°C. on a water bath. Add *B* to *A* slowly, stirring until congealed.

This smooth, medium-soft preparation spreads readily and can be removed quickly with water. Viscous liquids and powders, such as lanolin and zinc oxide, combine well with this base.

PADBASE

	grams
A. Cetyl Alcohol	13.000
White Petrolatum	10.000
White Beeswax	2.000
B. Glycerin	8.000
Sodium Lauryl Sulfate	1.000
Distilled Water	66.000
Methyl Paraben	0.015
Propyl Paraben	0.015

Heat *A* to 70°C. Heat *B* to 70°C. on a water bath. Add *B* to *A* slowly, stirring until congealed.

This smooth, white base spreads easily and has very good adhesive and absorbent character. It is practically greaseless and can be applied to large areas as a simple emollient or in combination with other dermatological agents. Resorcin and boric acid are incorporated satisfactorily in this vehicle.

CETOBASE

		grams
A.	Cetyl Alcohol	16.000
	Stearyl Alcohol	8.000
	White Petrolatum	26.000
B.	Glycerin	10.000
	Sodium Lauryl Sulfate	1.000
	Distilled Water	39.000
	Methyl Paraben	0.015
	Propyl Paraben	0.015

Heat *A* to 70°C. Heat *B* to 70°C. on a water bath. Add *B* to *A* slowly, stirring until congealed.

This yields a smooth, white, heavy-bodied base having good adhesive and absorbent properties. It is well suited for absorption of large amounts of liquid. Its removal is simple with water. It is especially useful with methyl salicylate and benzyl benzoate.

NORMABASE

		grams
A.	Stearic Acid	6.000
	Self-Emulsifying Glyceryl Monostearate	9.000
	White Petrolatum	21.000
	White Beeswax	4.000
B.	Sodium Lauryl Sulfate	0.500
	Glycerin	5.000
	Distilled Water	54.500
	Methyl Paraben	0.015
	Propyl Paraben	0.015

Heat *A* to 75°C. Heat *B* to 75°C. on a water bath. Add *B* to *A* slowly, stirring until congealed.

This smooth, heavy-bodied vehicle is suitable for general-purpose work, especially for the absorption of oily liquids. It is suggested for cod liver oil or methyl salicylate.

EFFBASE

		grams
A.	Stearic Acid	7.000
	Cetyl Alcohol	7.000
	White Petrolatum	24.000
B.	Sodium Lauryl Sulfate	1.000
	Distilled Water	61.000
	Methyl Paraben	0.015
	Propyl Paraben	0.015

Heat *A* to 75°C. Heat *B* to 75°C. on a water bath. Add *B* to *A* slowly, stirring until congealed.

This medium-bodied vehicle spreads well. It is suitable for use with powdered drugs. Sulfathiazole and bismuth subnitrate are easy to incorporate.

SANABASE

		grams
A.	Cetyl Alcohol	20.000
	White Petrolatum	30.000
	White Beeswax	1.000
B.	Glycerin	8.000
	Sodium Lauryl Sulfate	1.000
	Distilled Water	40.000
	Methyl Paraben	0.015
	Propyl Paraben	0.015

Heat *A* to 75°C. Heat *B* to 75°C. on a water bath. Add *A* to *B* slowly, stirring until congealed.

This firm, heavy-bodied base can serve as a medium for the absorption of a large volume of liquid medication. It is also suitable for use with light powders, such as salicylic or benzoic acid.

DESABASE

		grams
A.	Spermaceti	10.000
	Cetyl Alcohol	4.000
	White Petrolatum	18.000
	Liquid Petrolatum	9.000
B.	Sodium Lauryl Sulfate	1.000
	Distilled Water	58.000
	Methyl Paraben	0.015
	Propyl Paraben	0.015

Heat *A* to 70°C. Heat *B* to 70°C. on a water bath. Add *A* to *B* slowly, stirring until congealed.

This is a medium-bodied general-purpose unguent base. It can be applied or removed easily and is relatively greaseless. Calamine and resorcin combine very satisfactorily with this preparation.

IVABASE

		grams
A.	Self-Emulsifying Glyceryl Monostearate	10.000
	Spermaceti	9.000
	White Petrolatum	10.000
	Liquid Petrolatum	6.000
B.	Glycerin	6.000
	Distilled Water	59.000
	Methyl Paraben	0.015
	Propyl Paraben	0.015

Heat *A* to 70°C. Heat *B* to 70°C. on a water bath. Add *B* to *A* slowly, stirring until congealed.

This is a nonionic, medium-bodied vehicle for use as a simple emollient and protective. It is practically nongreasy and can, therefore, be applied to large areas comfortably. Additional medications can be included if desired. Ammoniated mercury incorporates very well in this base.

EMULSIBASE

		grams
A.	Stearyl Alcohol	12.000

	White Petrolatum	25.000
	Liquid Petrolatum	5.000
	White Beeswax	4.000
B.	Glycerin	6.000
	Sodium Lauryl Sulfate	1.000
	Distilled Water	47.000
	Methyl Paraben	0.015
	Propyl Paraben	0.015

Heat *A* to 70°C. Heat *B* to 70°C. on a water bath. Add *B* to *A* slowly, stirring until congealed.

This heavy-bodied vehicle has good adhesive and absorption character. It is best suited for the absorption of liquids and semisolids. Lanolin or crude coal tar produce a smooth, homogeneous unguent.

ROWBASE

		grams
A.	Stearic Acid	9.000
	Self-Emulsifying Glyceryl Monostearate	10.000
	Liquid Petrolatum	8.000
	White Beeswax	3.000
B.	Glycerin	4.000
	Distilled Water	66.000
	Methyl Paraben	0.015
	Propyl Paraben	0.015

Heat *A* to 75°C. Heat *B* to 75°C. on a water bath. Add *B* to *A* slowly, stirring until congealed.

This is a nonionic, smooth-spreading vehicle of medium body. It is quite greaseless and can be applied to large areas. Various therapeutic agents may be added. Powders are combined easily with this base. A good preparation is obtained with bismuth subgallate or calamine.

MELOBASE

		grams
A.	Cetyl Alcohol	7.000
	Self-Emulsifying Glyceryl Monostearate	7.000
	White Petrolatum	27.000

B.	Sodium Lauryl Sulfate	1.000
	Distilled Water	58.000
	Methyl Paraben	0.015
	Propyl Paraben	0.015

Heat *A* to 70°C. Heat *B* to 70°C. on a water bath. Add *B* to *A* slowly, stirring until congealed.

A smooth, firm, heavy-bodied base results which is suitable for general-purpose work. It is compatible with a large number of dermatological agents. Sulfur or cod-liver oil are easily incorporated.

DOLBASE

		grams
A.	Stearyl Alcohol	6.000
	Stearic Acid	2.000
	Cetyl Alcohol	4.000
	White Beeswax	2.000
	White Petrolatum	30.000
B.	Glycerin	5.000
	Sodium Lauryl Sulfate	1.000
	Distilled Water	50.000
	Methyl Paraben	0.015
	Propyl Paraben	0.015

Heat *A* to 75°C. Heat *B* to 75°C. on a water bath. Add *B* to *A* slowly, stirring until congealed.

This heavy-bodied vehicle has good adhesive character and is suitable for general-purpose work. It is compatible with powders and oily liquids. Sulfur or thymol iodide form a smooth unguent.

WHITBASE

		grams
A.	Self-Emulsifying Glyceryl Monostearate	9.000
	Stearyl Alcohol	4.000
	Cetyl Alcohol	7.000
	White Petrolatum	14.000
	White Beeswax	2.000
B.	Glycerin	4.000
	Distilled Water	60.000
	Methyl Paraben	0.015

Propyl Paraben	0.015

Heat *A* to 70°C. Heat *B* to 70°C. on a water bath. Add *B* to *A* slowly, stirring until congealed.

This greaseless, heavy-bodied nonionic base is adapted to general-purpose work. The majority of therapeutic agents can be incorporated with it. Aqueous and oily liquids, such as oil of cade or benzyl benzoate, are readily absorbed.

ADBASE

		grams
A.	Spermaceti	8.000
	Cetyl Alcohol	8.000
	White Petrolatum	12.000
	White Beeswax	2.000
B.	Glycerin	6.000
	Sodium Lauryl Sulfate	1.000
	Distilled Water	63.000
	Methyl Paraben	0.015
	Propyl Paraben	0.015

Heat *A* to 70°C. Heat *B* to 70°C. on a water bath. Add *B* to *A* slowly, stirring until congealed.

This smooth, soft, light-bodied vehicle spreads easily and can be applied over large areas as a greaseless emollient. Powdered dermatologic agents are best suited for use with this base. Calomel or oxyquinoline give a very satisfactory unguent.

ALBABASE

		grams
A.	Stearyl Alcohol	4.000
	Self-Emulsifying Glyceryl Monostearate	10.000
	White Petrolatum	14.000
B.	Glycerin	4.000
	Distilled Water	68.000
	Methyl Paraben	0.015
	Propyl Paraben	0.015

Heat *A* to 70°C. Heat *B* to 70°C. on a water bath. Add *B* to *A* slowly, stirring until congealed.

This yields a smooth, nonionic, medium-bodied preparation which is suitable for general-purpose work. Most dermatologic agents are compatible with this base which is greaseless and spreads evenly in thin layers. Phenol or zinc oxide are readily incorporated to form a good unguent. It absorbs powders and oily liquids.

IRABASE

		grams
A.	Cetyl Alcohol	13.000
	White Beeswax	2.000
B.	Glycerin	6.000
	Sodium Lauryl Sulfate	1.000
	Distilled Water	78.000
	Methyl Paraben	0.015
	Propyl Paraben	0.015

Heat *A* to 70°C. Heat *B* to 70°C. on a water bath. Add *B* to *A* slowly, stirring until congealed.

This soft, light-bodied preparation can be applied easily to large areas. It is nongreasy and can be removed quickly with water. Powders and oily liquids, such as starch or sulfonated castor oil, are best suited for this vehicle.

DILUBASE

		grams
A.	Self-Emulsifying Glyceryl Monostearate	9.000
	Spermaceti	15.000
	Span 60*	6.000
B.	Tween 40*	4.000
	Glycerin	6.000
	Distilled Water	60.000
	Methyl Paraben	0.015
	Propyl Paraben	0.015

Heat *A* to 70°C. Heat *B* to 70°C. on a water bath. Add *B* to *A* slowly, stirring until congealed.

This nonionic, soft-bodied preparation can be applied to large areas. It is best suited for incorporation with powdered medicinal agents. Ammoniated mercury or resorcin combines very easily with this base.

*Atlas Powder Co.

PROPABASE

		grams
A.	Stearic Acid	12.000
	Stearyl Alcohol	12.000
	White Petrolatum	12.000
	White Beeswax	4.000
	Liquid Petrolatum	5.000
B.	Glycerin	4.000
	Sodium Lauryl Sulfate	1.000
	Distilled Water	50.000
	Methyl Paraben	0.015
	Propyl Paraben	0.015

Heat *A* to 75°C. Heat *B* to 75°C. on a water bath. Add *B* to *A* slowly, stirring until congealed.

This is a smooth-textured, adhesive base of medium-heavy body. It is suitable for general-purpose work and especially for liquid absorption. It is relatively nongreasy and spreads evenly. Alcoholic solutions, e.g., of coal tar, are easy to incorporate.

DOEBASE

		grams
A.	Stearyl Alcohol	10.000
	Cetyl Alcohol	9.000
	White Beeswax	2.000
	Span 60*	9.000
B.	Tween 40*	5.000
	Distilled Water	65.000
	Methyl Paraben	0.015
	Propyl Paraben	0.015

Heat *A* to 85°C. Heat *B* to 85°C. on a water bath. Add *B* to *A* slowly, stirring until congealed.

This greaseless, nonionic, heavy-bodied base is excellent for liquid absorption. It can also be used with all other groups of therapeutic agents. It takes up readily benzyl benzoate or methyl salicylate.

---

*Atlas Powder Co.

GEOBASE

		grams
A.	Cetyl Alcohol	10.000
	White Petrolatum	23.000
	Liquid Petrolatum	7.000
	White Beeswax	4.000
B.	Glycerin	5.000
	Sodium Lauryl Sulfate	1.000
	Distilled Water	50.000
	Methyl Paraben	0.015
	Propyl Paraben	0.015

Heat *A* to 70°C. Heat *B* to 70°C. on a water bath. Add *B* to *A* slowly, stirring until congealed.

This medium-bodied base has good adhesive and spreading properties. It is best suited for use with oily and viscous liquids, such as crude coal tar or balsam of Peru.

TUABASE

		grams
A.	Self-Emulsifying Glyceryl Monostearate	15.000
	White Petrolatum	20.000
	Liquid Petrolatum	3.000
	White Beeswax	2.000
B.	Glycerin	7.000
	Distilled Water	53.000
	Methyl Paraben	0.015
	Propyl Paraben	0.015

Heat *A* to 70°C. Heat *B* to 70°C. on a water bath. Add *B* to *A* slowly, stirring until congealed.

This is a good, general-purpose base of the nonionic type. It is compatible with most dermatological agents and has satisfactory liquid absorption properties. Ichthammol or ammoniated mercury combine very well with this preparation.

DEMIBASE

		grams
A.	Stearyl Alcohol	18.000

B.	Glycerin	6.000
	Sodium Lauryl Sulfate	1.000
	Distilled Water	75.000
	Methyl Paraben	0.015
	Propyl Paraben	0.015

Heat *A* to 70°C. Heat *B* to 70°C. on a water bath. Add *B* to *A* slowly, stirring until congealed.

This smooth, medium-bodied, absorptive vehicle is suitable for general-purpose work. Without medication, it will serve as a good emollient and protective agent. Tannic acid or a solution of coal tar can be very well incorporated.

TONABASE

		grams
A.	Cetyl Alcohol	18.000
	White Petrolatum	18.000
B.	Glycerin	6.000
	Sodium Lauryl Sulfate	1.000
	Distilled Water	57.000
	Methyl Paraben	0.015
	Propyl Paraben	0.015

Heat *A* to 70°C. Heat *B* to 70°C. on a water bath. Add *A* to *B* slowly, stirring until congealed.

This is a very good, medium-bodied absorptive base of fine texture. It is quite greaseless and can be removed easily with water. Most dermatologic agents are compatible with it. Ichthammol or tannic acid produces a smooth unguent with this vehicle.

JERIBASE

		grams
A.	Stearic Acid	8.000
	Spermaceti	10.000
	Cetyl Alcohol	5.000
	White Petrolatum	20.000
	Liquid Petrolatum	5.000
B.	Sodium Lauryl Sulfate	1.000
	Distilled Water	51.000

Methyl Paraben	0.015
Propyl Paraben	0.015

Heat *A* to 75°C. Heat *B* to 75°C. on a water bath. Add *A* to *B* slowly, stirring until congealed.

This is a very smooth, heavy-bodied vehicle which spreads easily and rinses off quickly with water. It is suitable for general-purpose work. Olive oil or methyl salicylate combines easily with it to form a satisfactory unguent.

WELBASE

	grams
Self-Emulsifying Glyceryl Monostearate	21.000
White Petrolatum	22.000
Distilled Water	57.000
Methyl Paraben	0.015
Propyl Paraben	0.015

Heat all together to 70°C. on a water bath. Stir slowly until congealed.

This is a firm, heavy-bodied preparation of the nonionic class. It is suitable for use with all types of medication. It absorbs liquids, such as boric acid solution or rose water very easily.

TRUBASE

		grams
A.	Spermaceti	5.000
	Self-Emulsifying Glyceryl Monostearate	10.000
	Liquid Petrolatum	21.000
	White Petrolatum	7.000
B.	Propylene Glycol	7.000
	Distilled Water	50.000
	Methyl Paraben	0.015
	Propyl Paraben	0.015

Heat *A* to 70°C. Heat *B* to 70°C. on a water bath. Add *B* to *A* slowly, stirring until congealed.

This nonionic, greaseless, medium-bodied base can be combined with all types of therapeutic agents. It can be applied or removed easily and is very useful for general-purpose work. Powdered drugs, such as precipitated sulfur or salicylic acid are suitable for combination with this vehicle.

EUROBASE

	grams
A. Stearyl Alcohol	24.000
Liquid Petrolatum	10.000
White Beeswax	6.000
B. Sodium Lauryl Sulfate	1.000
Distilled Water	59.000
Methyl Paraben	0.015
Propyl Paraben	0.015

Heat *A* to 70°C. Heat *B* to 70°C. on a water bath. Add *A* to *B* slowly, stirring until congealed.

This firm, smooth, heavy-bodied base is useful for incorporation with oily liquids and semisolids. It spreads evenly and has good absorbent properties. Lanolin or balsam of Peru combine well with this preparation.

SIRBASE

	grams
A. Stearic Acid	13.000
Cetyl Alcohol	5.000
Liquid Petrolatum	20.000
B. Glycerin	3.000
Sodium Lauryl Sulfate	1.000
Distilled Water	58.000
Methyl Paraben	0.015
Propyl Paraben	0.015

Heat *A* to 75°C. Heat *B* to 75°C. on a water bath. Add *B* to *A* slowly, stirring until congealed.

This is a smooth, nongreasy, general-purpose vehicle of medium body. It is especially useful for powdered medicinal agents, such as boric acid or bismuth subgallate.

WINBASE

	grams
Self-Emulsifying Glyceryl Monostearate	14.000
White Petrolatum	26.000
Liquid Petrolatum	11.000
Distilled Water	45.000
Methyl Paraben	0.015
Propyl Paraben	0.015

Heat all together to 70 °C. on a water bath. Stir slowly, until congealed.

A medium-bodied nonionic preparation is obtained that can be used with all types of medication. It has good liquid absorbent character and combines with oil of cade or crude coal tar readily to form a smooth-textured unguent.

MONBASE

	grams
A. Stearyl Alcohol	23.000
White Petrolatum	32.000
B. Glycerin	10.000
Sodium Lauryl Sulfate	1.000
Distilled Water	34.000
Methyl Paraben	0.015
Propyl Paraben	0.015

Heat *A* to 75 °C. Heat *B* to 75 °C. on a water bath. Add *B* to *A* slowly, stirring until congealed.

This adhesive, heavy-bodied base shows very good liquid absorption. Most dermatologic agents in liquid or powdered form can be easily added. Camphor, menthol, or salicylic acid yield a fine-textured unguent.

NUBASE

	grams
Stearic Acid	15.000
Cetyl Alcohol	2.000
Self-Emulsifying Glyceryl Monostearate	5.000

White Petrolatum	24.000
Span 60*	4.000
Tween 40*	2.000
Distilled Water	48.000
Methyl Paraben	0.015
Propyl Paraben	0.015

Heat all together to 80°C. on a water bath. Stir slowly until congealed.

This nonionic, heavy-bodied preparation is quite greaseless and compatible with all classes of therapeutic agents. It absorbs large volumes of liquids, such as copper sulfate or sodium thiosulfate solutions.

*Atlas Powder Co.

DEKABASE

		grams
A.	Spermaceti	10.000
	Cetyl Alcohol	7.000
	White Beeswax	2.000
	White Petrolatum	8.000
B.	Glycerin	6.000
	Sodium Lauryl Sulfate	1.000
	Distilled Water	66.000
	Methyl Paraben	0.015
	Propyl Paraben	0.015

Heat *A* to 70°C. Heat *B* to 70°C. on a water bath. Add *B* to *A* slowly, stirring until congealed.

This soft, light-bodied base is suitable for spreading on large areas. Powdered or semisolid medicaments are best incorporated. Lanolin or bismuth subnitrate forms a smooth homogeneous unguent.

Chapter Three

WASHABLE OIL-IN-WATER LOTIONS

TEMPLOTION

		grams
A.	Stearyl Alcohol	3.750
	White Beeswax	0.500
	Span 60*	1.750
B.	Tween 40*	1.000
	Distilled Water	93.000
	Methyl Paraben	0.015
	Propyl Paraben	0.015

Heat *A* to 85°C. Heat *B* to 85°C. on a water bath. Add *B* to *A* slowly, stirring until it cools to 40°C.

This nonionic, light-bodied lotion is suitable for general-purpose work. It is compatible with the majority of dermatological agents. It is especially well suited for use with oily liquids, such as benzyl benzoate.

*Atlas Powder Co.

MELOLOTION

		grams
A.	Spermaceti	3.000
	Liquid Petrolatum	3.000
B.	Sodium Lauryl Sulfate	1.000
	Distilled Water	93.000
	Methyl Paraben	0.015
	Propyl Paraben	0.015

Heat *A* to 70°C. Heat *B* to 70°C. on a water bath. Add *B* to *A* slowly, stirring until it cools to 40°C.

This is a pleasing, light-bodied vehicle which is easily incorporated with the majority of dermatological agents. It is free flowing for use on large areas. It is easy to combine with aqueous liquids and powdered drugs, such as lime water, tannic acid, phenol, or lead subacetate solution.

SOLALOTION

		grams
A.	Cetyl Alcohol	1.000
	Self-Emulsifying Glyceryl Monostearate	2.250
	White Beeswax	0.500
	White Petrolatum	9.500
B.	Glycerin	1.000
	Distilled Water	85.750
	Methyl Paraben	0.015
	Propyl Paraben	0.015

Heat *A* to 70°C. Heat *B* to 70°C. on a water bath. Add *B* to *A* slowly, stirring until it cools to 35°C.

This is a smooth, white, nonionic lotion of medium viscosity. It flows freely and is relatively nongreasy. It combines easily with the most common drugs, both in liquid and powder form. Phenol and Burow's solution are especially well taken up by this lotion.

FINLOTION

		grams
A.	Stearyl Alcohol	2.000
	Cetyl Alcohol	1.000
	White Petrolatum	5.750
	Liquid Petrolatum	2.250
B.	Sodium Lauryl Sulfate	0.250
	Distilled Water	88.750
	Methyl Paraben	0.015
	Propyl Paraben	0.015

Heat A to 70°C. Heat *B* to 70°C. on a water bath. Add *B* to *A* slowly, stirring until it cools to 35°C.

This free-flowing, medium-bodied lotion can be used for general-purpose work. It is comparatively greaseless and is readily removed with water. Aqueous or alcoholic liquids, such as solutions of sodium thiosulfate are quite compatible with this vehicle.

IVILOTION

		grams
A.	Cetyl Alcohol	2.600
	White Petrolatum	2.000
	White Beeswax	0.400
B.	Glycerin	1.600
	Sodium Lauryl Sulfate	0.200
	Distilled Water	93.200
	Methyl Paraben	0.015
	Propyl Paraben	0.015

Heat *A* to 70°C. Heat *B* to 70°C. on a water bath. Add *B* to *A* slowly, stirring until it cools to 35°C.

This white, light-bodied vehicle can be used on large areas without discomfort. Alone, it will serve as a protective agent. It is especially suitable for aqueous or alcoholic solutions, such as Burow's solution and solutions of coal tar.

LOFTLOTION

		grams
A.	Stearic Acid	1.500
	Stearyl Alcohol	1.500
	Liquid Petrolatum	22.000
B.	Glycerin	2.000
	Sodium Lauryl Sulfate	1.000
	Distilled Water	72.000
	Methyl Paraben	0.015
	Propyl Paraben	0.015

Heat *A* to 75°C. Heat *B* to 75°C. on a water bath. Add *B* to *A* slowly, stirring until it cools to 40°C.

This well-balanced, medium-bodied lotion has excellent lubricating properties. It flows easily, adheres well, and rinses off quickly with water. It combines with a large number of dermatological agents.

Used alone, it is an effective lubricant. Oily, aqueous, and alcoholic liquids, e.g., pyrogallol, Burow's solution and tincture of capsicum, can be easily incorporated.

EDYLOTION

	grams
Self-Emulsifying Glyceryl Monostearate	4.200
White Petrolatum	4.400
Distilled Water	91.400
Methyl Paraben	0.015
Propyl Paraben	0.015

Heat all together to 70°C. on a water bath. Stir slowly until it cools to 35°C.

This is a nonionic, homogeneous lotion of the nonionic type. It is compatible with practically all medicinal agents. It flows freely and spreads easily. It is suitable for general-purpose work, but better adapted to combination with substances in liquid form. Solutions of coal tar and potassium iodide are equally well absorbed to yield a homogeneous product.

PERRILOTION

		grams
A.	Stearyl Alcohol	1.800
	Cetyl Alcohol	2.400
	White Petrolatum	5.600
B.	Propylene Glycol	1.600
	Sodium Lauryl Sulfate	0.200
	Distilled Water	88.400
	Methyl Paraben	0.015
	Propyl Paraben	0.015

Heat *A* to 70°C. Heat *B* to 70°C. on a water bath. Add *B* to *A* slowly, stirring until it cools to 35°C.

This homogeneous, medium-bodied lotion is easily applied or removed. It is especially good for use with liquids, such as cod-liver oil.

DURALOTION

		grams
A.	Self-Emsulsifying Glyceryl Monostearate	3.200

Stearyl Alcohol	1.400
White Beeswax	0.400
White Petrolatum	1.200
B. Glycerin	0.800
Distilled Water	93.000
Methyl Paraben	0.015
Propyl Paraben	0.015

Heat *A* to 70°C. Heat *B* to 70°C. on a water bath. Add *B* to *A* slowly, stirring until it cools to 35°C.

This homogeneous, heavy-bodied lotion can be used with larger volumes of liquid medicinal agents. It pours and spreads readily, and is rinsed off with water. Lime water or copper sulfate solution can be incorporated to form a satisfactory lotion.

SURFALOTION

	grams
A. Stearic Acid	1.750
Cetyl Alcohol	2.000
White Petrolatum	6.000
B. Sodium Lauryl Sulfate	0.250
Distilled Water	90.000
Methyl Paraben	0.015
Propyl Paraben	0.015

Heat *A* to 75°C. Heat *B* to 75°C. on a water bath. Add *B* to *A* slowly, stirring until it cools to 35°C.

This fine, light-bodied lotion flows freely and washes off easily. Bismuth subgallate and magnesium oxide combine with it to form a satisfactory lotion. Powdered drugs can also be used with this vehicle.

NATALOTION

	grams
Liquid Petrolatum	3.500
Self-Emulsifying Glyceryl Monostearate	2.500
Distilled Water	94.000
Methyl Paraben	0.015
Propyl Paraben	0.015

Heat all together to 70°C. on a water bath. Slowly stir until it cools to 40°C.

This pleasant, nonionic, light-bodied, washable lotion flows freely and spreads readily. It is compatible with all kinds of medicinal agents. It combines very well with aqueous and powdered drugs, such as camphor water, boric acid solution, or zinc oxide.

AGUALOTION

		grams
A.	Cetyl Alcohol	4.350
	White Beeswax	1.000
B.	Glycerin	2.300
	Sodium Lauryl Sulfate	0.350
	Distilled Water	92.000
	Methyl Paraben	0.015
	Propyl Paraben	0.015

Heat *A* to 70°C. Heat *B* to 70°C. on a water bath. Add *B* to *A* slowly, stirring until it cools to 35°C.

This smooth, heavy-bodied lotion has good adhesive and spreading character. It absorbs aqueous or alcoholic liquids, such as camphor water or coal tar solutions.

GENTILOTION

		grams
A.	Stearic Acid	0.500
	Stearyl Alcohol	1.500
	Cetyl Alcohol	1.000
	White Beeswax	0.500
	White Petrolatum	7.500
B.	Glycerin	1.250
	Sodium Lauryl Sulfate	0.250
	Distilled Water	87.500
	Methyl Paraben	0.015
	Propyl Paraben	0.015

Heat *A* to 75°C. Heat *B* to 75°C. on a water bath. Add *B* to *A* slowly, stirring until it cools to 35°C.

This homogeneous, light-bodied, washable vehicle flows freely and is compatible with a large number of medicinal agents. Powders and oily liquids, such as olive oil or calamine, combine well with this lotion.

MAJORLOTION

		grams
A.	Self-Emulsifying Glyceryl Monostearate	2.500
	Cetyl Alcohol	0.850
	White Petrolatum	2.500
	White Beeswax	0.500
B.	Glycerin	1.150
	Distilled Water	92.500
	Methyl Paraben	0.015
	Propyl Paraben	0.015

Heat *A* to 70°C. Heat *B* to 70°C. on a water bath. Add *B* to *A* slowly, stirring until it cools to 35°C.

This is a smooth, white, light-bodied lotion of the nonionic group. It combines easily with a large number of dermatological agents. It is especially useful with powders, such as zinc oxide or talc.

PARALOTION

		grams
A.	Stearic Acid	1.250
	Cetyl Alcohol	1.500
	White Beeswax	0.750
	White Petrolatum	7.000
B.	Glycerin	2.000
	Sodium Lauryl Sulfate	0.250
	Distilled Water	87.250
	Methyl Paraben	0.015
	Propyl Paraben	0.015

Heat *A* to 75°C. Heat *B* to 75°C. on a water bath. Add *B* to *A* slowly, stirring until it cools to 35°C.

This free-flowing, medium-bodied vehicle is suitable for general-purpose use. Methyl salicylate and other essential oils show good compatibility with this lotion.

MISTLOTION

	grams
A. Stearyl Alcohol	6.000
Liquid Petrolatum	2.500
White Beeswax	1.500
Sodium Lauryl Sulfate	0.250
B. Distilled Water	89.750
Methyl Paraben	0.015
Propyl Paraben	0.015

Heat *A* to 70°C. Heat *B* to 70°C. on a water bath. Add *B* to *A* slowly, stirring until it cools to 35°C.

This smooth, medium-bodied lotion is suitable as a simple emollient or as a vehicle for oily liquids, such as olive oil or methyl salicylate. It flows easily and washes readily with water.

PROVOLOTION

	grams
A. Self-Emulsifying Glyceryl Monostearate	2.250
Stearyl Alcohol	1.000
Cetyl Alcohol	1.750
White Petrolatum	3.500
White Beeswax	0.500
B. Glycerin	1.000
Distilled Water	90.000
Methyl Paraben	0.015
Propyl Paraben	0.015

Heat *A* to 70°C. Heat *B* to 70°C. on a water bath. Add *B* to *A* slowly, stirring until it cools to 35°C.

This smooth easy-flowing, heavy-bodied lotion belongs to the non-ionic group. It combines with most types of medication and is practically nongrease. It is suitable for use with aqueous or alcoholic liquids, such as rose water and tinctures.

ROSALOTION

	grams
A. Cetyl Alcohol	2.500

White Petrolatum	5.750
Liquid Petrolatum	1.750
White Beeswax	1.000
B. Glycerin	1.250
Sodium Lauryl Sulfate	0.250
Distilled Water	87.500
Methyl Paraben	0.015
Propyl Paraben	0.015

Heat *A* to 70°C. Heat *B* to 70°C. on a water bath. Add *B* to *A* slowly, stirring until it cools to 35°C.

This smooth, light-bodied vehicle can be applied to large areas. It flows freely and can be removed easily with water. Alcoholic or oily liquids, such as tincture of benzoin or resorcin monoacetate, combine well forming a good homogeneous lotion.

TECTILOTION

	grams
A. Stearyl Alcohol	4.000
Liquid Petrolatum	18.000
White Beeswax	1.000
B. Sodium Lauryl Sulfate	1.000
Distilled Water	76.000
Methyl Paraben	0.015
Propyl Paraben	0.015

Heat *A* to 70°C. Heat *B* to 70°C. on a water bath. Add *B* to *A* slowly, stirring until it cools to 40°C.

This smooth, medium-bodied vehicle adheres well and is a good emollient. It is free flowing, spreads easily, and is washable. Because of its wide range of compatibility, it is well suited for general-purpose work. Powdered drugs, such as bismuth subgallate or salicylic acid, combine very well with this lotion.

SEDLOTION

	grams
A. Spermaceti	2.650
Cetyl Alcohol	2.650
White Petrolatum	4.000

	White Beeswax	0.650
B.	Glycerin	1.700
	Sodium Lauryl Sulfate	0.350
	Distilled Water	88.000
	Methyl Paraben	0.015
	Propyl Paraben	0.015

Heat *A* to 70°C. Heat *B* to 70°C. on a water bath. Add *B* to *A* slowly, stirring until it cools to 35°C.

This light-bodied, nongreasy, washable lotion flows freely and spreads easily. Oily liquids and light powders are easily incorporated. Resorcin or castor oil combines well with this vehicle.

MONALOTION

	grams
Self-Emulsifying Glyceryl Monostearate	4.000
Glycerin	3.000
Beeswax	0.500
Distilled Water	92.500
Methyl Paraben	0.015
Propyl Paraben	0.015

Heat all together to 70°C. on a water bath. Stir slowly until it cools to 35°C.

This smooth, light-bodied, nonionic lotion is compatible with the majority of therapeutic agents. It can be employed on large areas alone as an emollient or in combination with oily liquids or powders. Almond oil, cod-liver oil, or tannic acid will give a satisfactory lotion.

FELDLOTION

		grams
A.	Stearyl Alcohol	1.000
	Cetyl Alcohol	2.350
	White Beeswax	1.300
	White Petrolatum	9.000
B.	Glycerin	2.500
	Sodium Lauryl Sulfate	0.350
	Distilled Water	83.500
	Methyl Paraben	0.015

Propyl Paraben	0.015

Heat *A* to 70°C. Heat *B* to 70°C. on a water bath. Add *B* to *A* slowly, stirring until it cools to 35°C.

This homogeneous, medium-bodied, washable vehicle can be combined with the majority of therapeutic agents, such as magnesium oxide or methyl salicylate, or used alone as an emollient.

MARMALOTION

	grams
A. Cetyl Alcohol	2.500
Stearic Acid	0.500
B. Glycerin	8.000
Sodium Lauryl Sulfate	1.000
Distilled Water	88.000
Methyl Paraben	0.015
Propyl Paraben	0.015

Heat *A* to 75°C. Heat *B* to 75°C. on a water bath. Add *B* to *A* slowly, stirring until it cools to 40°C.

This is a free-flowing, light-bodied preparation for general-purpose use. It is especially well adapted for combination with oily and alcoholic liquids, such as olive oil or solutions of coal tar. It can be easily washed off with water from the skin.

SPRILOTION

	grams
Self-Emulsifying Glyceryl Monostearate	2.000
Stearic Acid	1.250
White Petrolatum	8.750
Distilled Water	88.000
Methyl Paraben	0.015
Propyl Paraben	0.015

Heat all together to 75°C. on a water bath. Stir slowly until it cools to 35°C.

This greaseless nonionic lotion can be combined with all types of medicinal substances. It is of medium consistency, pours freely, and spreads easily. It is suitable for use with such liquids as *Liquor Carbonis Detergens*.

SIDROLOTION

		grams
A.	Cetyl Alcohol	2.000
	Stearic Acid	1.000
	Liquid Petrolatum	22.000
	White Beeswax	2.000
B.	Glycerin	3.000
	Sodium Lauryl Sulfate	1.000
	Distilled Water	69.000
	Methyl Paraben	0.015
	Propyl Paraben	0.015

Heat *A* to 75°C. Heat *B* to 75°C. on a water bath. Add *B* to *A* slowly, stirring until it cools to 40°C.

This well-balanced lotion of medium body flows readily, spreads easily, and washes quickly with water. Most medicinal agents will combine well with this vehicle. It has a high degree of emollient action due to a greater than usual oil content. It absorbs aqueous liquids and powdered drugs, such as Burow's solution, resorcin, or boric acid.

ERGOLOTION

		grams
A.	Spermaceti	1.000
	Stearyl Alcohol	4.000
	White Petrolatum	5.800
B.	Glycerin	2.000
	Sodium Lauryl Sulfate	0.200
	Distilled Water	87.000
	Methyl Paraben	0.015
	Propyl Paraben	0.015

Heat *A* to 70°C. Heat *B* to 70°C. on a water bath. Add *B* to *A* slowly, stirring until it cools to 35°C.

This viscous, heavy-bodied, washable lotion has good adhesive and covering character. It is especially useful in combination with liquid dermatological agents. Resorcin and resorcin monoacetate (Euresol) are compatible with this lotion.

NEETLOTION

	grams
Self-Emulsifying Glyceryl Monostearate	4.000
Liquid Petrolatum	10.000
White Beeswax	2.000
Distilled Water	84.000
Methyl Paraben	0.015
Propyl Paraben	0.015

Heat all together to 70°C. on a water bath. Stir slowly until it cools to 40°C.

This is a homogeneous nonionic lotion of medium body. It has a very high degree of drug compatibility. It flows and spreads readily. Without medication, it serves as an excellent emollient and protective agent. It absorbs powders, such as sulfur, talc, and oxyquinolines.

PORTLOTION

		grams
A.	Cetyl Alcohol	3.250
	White Beeswax	0.500
B.	Glycerin	1.500
	Sodium Lauryl Sulfate	0.250
	Distilled Water	94.500
	Methyl Paraben	0.015
	Propyl Paraben	0.015

Heat *A* to 70°C. Heat *B* to 70°C. on a water bath. Add *B* to *A* slowly, stirring until it cools to 35°C.

This homogeneous, light-bodied vehicle is greaseless and free flowing. It takes up liquids and powders alike, e.g., tannic acid or magnesium oxide.

ELILOTION

	grams
Self-Emulsifying Glyceryl Monostearate	4.250
White Petrolatum	4.750
Distilled Water	91.000
Methyl Paraben	0.015
Propyl Paraben	0.015

Heat all together to 70°C. on a water bath. Stir slowly until it cools to 35°C.

This pleasant, easily-applied lotion of medium body serves as a good, general-purpose vehicle. It is relatively nongreasy and readily removable. It can be used with phenol.

CLYMALOTION

		grams
A.	Stearic Acid	0.500
	Self-Emulsifying Glyceryl Monostearate	1.000
	Cetyl Alcohol	1.000
	White Beeswax	0.500
	White Petrolatum	4.000
B.	Glycerin	1.750
	Sodium Lauryl Sulfate	0.250
	Distilled Water	91.000
	Methyl Paraben	0.015
	Propyl Paraben	0.015

Heat *A* to 70°C. Heat *B* to 70°C. on a water bath. Add *B* to *A* slowly, stirring until it cools to 35°C.

This homogeneous, light-bodied vehicle flows freely and can be applied to large areas easily. Powdered therapeutic agents, such as starch or talc, are incorporated readily.

CETILOTION

		grams
A.	Spermacceti	1.250
	Cetyl Alcohol	1.750
	Stearyl Alcohol	0.750
	White Petrolatum	4.250
	Liquid Petrolatum	2.250
B.	Sodium Lauryl Sulfate	0.250
	Distilled Water	87.000
	Methyl Paraben	0.015
	Propyl Paraben	0.015

Heat *A* to 70°C. Heat *B* to 70°C. on a water bath. Add *B* to *A* slowly, stirring until it cools to 35°C.

This smooth, light-bodied lotion flows freely and can be spread easily and quickly over large areas. It is quite greaseless and may be combined with both liquid and powdered therapeutic agents, such as olive oil or boric acid solution.

SEPTALOTION

		grams
A.	Stearyl Alcohol	1.250
	Spermaceti	2.000
	Self-Emulsifying Glyceryl Monostearate	1.250
	White Petrolatum	5.500
	Span 40*	2.000
B.	Tween 40*	1.000
	Distilled Water	87.000
	Methyl Paraben	0.015
	Propyl Paraben	0.015

Heat *A* to 80°C. Heat *B* to 80°C. on a water bath. Add *B* to *A* slowly, stirring until it cools to 35°C.

This smooth, medium-bodied nonionic lotion is very useful for general-purpose work because of its compatibility with most medicaments. It flows easily and can be rinsed off quickly with water. Liquid or powdered drugs may be incorporated, such as balsam of Peru or phenol.

*Atlas Powder Co.

DEACLOTION

		grams
A.	Cetyl Alcohol	3.600
	White Petrolatum	3.600
B.	Glycerin	1.200
	Sodium Lauryl Sulfate	0.200
	Distilled Water	91.400
	Methyl Paraben	0.015
	Propyl Paraben	0.015

Heat *A* to 70°C. Heat *B* to 70°C. on a water bath. Add *B* to *A* slowly, stirring until it cools to 35°C.

This smooth, heavy-bodied vehicle adheres and spreads well. It can be combined with most dermatologic agents but is especially adapted for use with liquids, such as Burow's solution or lime water.

PELULOTION

		grams
A.	Stearic Acid	8.000
	White Beeswax	1.500
	Span 60*	4.000
B.	Tween 40*	4.000
	Distilled Water	82.500
	Methyl Paraben	0.015
	Propyl Paraben	0.015

Heat *A* to 85°C. Heat *B* to 85°C. on a water bath. Add *B* to *A* slowly, stirring until it cools to 35°C.

This very light-bodied lotion of the nonionic type is compatible with all groups of therapeutic agents. It flows freely and can be washed off quickly. Magnesium oxide or calamine combines very well.

*Atlas Powder Co.

ORTHOLOTION

		grams
A.	Self-Emulsifying Glyceryl Monostearate	1.250
	Cetyl Alcohol	1.250
	Stearyl Alcohol	1.250
	White Beeswax	0.500
	White Petrolatum	7.250
B.	Glycerin	1.250
	Sodium Lauryl Sulfate	0.250
	Distilled Water	87.000
	Methyl Paraben	0.015
	Propyl Paraben	0.015

Heat *A* to 70°C. Heat *B* to 70°C. on a water bath. Add *B* to *A* slowly, stirring until it cools to 35°C.

This good, medium-bodied lotion is suitable for general-purpose work. It flows freely and spreads easily. Oily liquids, such as methyl salicylate, incorporate very easily.

GENALOTION

		grams
A.	Stearic Acid	3.250
	Cetyl Alcohol	1.250
	Liquid Petrolatum	5.000
B.	Glycerin	0.750
	Sodium Lauryl Sulfate	0.250
	Distilled Water	89.500
	Methyl Paraben	0.015
	Propyl Paraben	0.015

Heat *A* to 75°C. Heat *B* to 75°C. on a water bath. Add *B* to *A* slowly, stirring until it cools to 35°C.

This homogeneous, light-bodied preparation flows and spreads easily. It can be used for general-purpose work or as a simple emollient. Powdered medicinal agents, such as zinc oxide or benzocaine, are absorbed very well.

THERALOTION

		grams
A.	Spermaceti	1.650
	Self-Emulsifying Glyceryl Monostearate	3.350
	Liquid Petrolatum	7.000
	White Petrolatum	2.350
B.	Proplylen Glycol	2.650
	Distilled Water	83.000
	Methyl Paraben	0.015
	Propyl Paraben	0.015

Heat *A* to 70°C. Heat *B* to 70°C. on a water bath. Add *B* to *A* slowly, stirring until it cools to 35°C.

This is a smooth, nonionic lotion of medium body. It spreads readily. Most medicinal agents, such as camphor, menthol, and phenol, are compatible with it.

BESSLOTION

		grams
A.	Stearic Acid	2.000
	Spermaceti	2.500

	Cetyl Alcohol	1.250
	White Petrolatum	5.000
	Liquid Petrolatum	1.250
B.	Sodium Lauryl Sulfate	0.250
	Distilled Water	87.750
	Methyl Paraben	0.015
	Propyl Paraben	0.015

Heat *A* to 75°C. Heat *B* to 75°C. on a water bath. Add *B* to *A* slowly, stirring until it cools to 35°C.

This smooth preparation of medium body is useful for general-purpose work. It flows and spreads readily. Without medication it is an effective emollient or protective. Tincture of benzoin or cod-liver oil produce a good lotion with this vehicle.

SELFLOTION

		grams
A.	Stearyl Alcohol	4.500
B.	Glycerin	1.500
	Sodium Lauryl Sulfate	0.250
	Distilled Water	93.750
	Methyl Paraben	0.015
	Propyl Paraben	0.015

Heat *A* to 70°C. Heat *B* to 70°C. on a water bath. Add *B* to *A* slowly, stirring until it cools to 35°C.

This smooth, heavy-bodied vehicle is suitable for general-purpose work and especially for combination with liquids, such as witch hazel or copper sulfate solution.

OBORLOTION

		grams
A.	Liquid Petrolatum	20.500
	Stearic Acid	6.500
B.	Glycerin	4.000
	Sodium Lauryl Sulfate	1.000
	Distilled Water	68.000
	Methyl Paraben	0.015
	Propyl Paraben	0.015

Heat *A* to 75°C. Heat *B* to 75°C. on a water bath. Add *B* to *A* slowly, stirring until it cools to 40°C.

This is a fine, smooth, adhesive lotion of medium body. It can serve as an efficient vehicle for all types of therapeutic agents, especially alcoholic and oily liquids, such as solutions of coal tar, tincture of benzoin, or solutions of phenol.

THANLOTION

		grams
A.	Cetyl Alcohol	2.600
	White Petrolatum	5.400
	White Beeswax	0.400
B.	Propylene Glycol	1.400
	Sodium Lauryl Sulfate	0.200
	Distilled Water	90.000
	Methyl Paraben	0.015
	Propyl Paraben	0.015

Heat *A* to 70°C. Heat *B* to 70°C. on a water bath. Add *B* to *A* slowly, stirring until it cools to 35°C.

This light, free-flowing preparation is compatible with a wide range of therapeutic agents. It is nongreasy and washable. Zinc oxide or calamine produces a good preparation with this lotion.

KESTILOTION

	grams
Self-Emulsifying Glyceryl Monostearate	3.500
White Petrolatum	6.500
Liquid Petrolatum	2.750
Distilled Water	86.250
Methyl Paraben	0.015
Propyl Paraben	0.015

Heat all together to 75°C. on a water bath. Stir slowly until it cools to 35°C.

This nonionic, medium-bodied, absorptive vehicle combines well with most dermatological agents. It can be applied or removed quickly. Precipitated sulfur or resorcin forms a smooth homogeneous suspension with this lotion.

TRAMLOTION

		grams
A.	Stearyl Alcohol	1.800
	Cetyl Alcohol	1.600
	White Petrolatum	2.600
	White Beeswax	0.400
B.	Propylene Glycol	1.400
	Sodium Lauryl Sulfate	0.200
	Distilled Water	92.000
	Methyl Paraben	0.015
	Propyl Paraben	0.015

Heat *A* to 70°C. Heat *B* to 70°C. on a water bath. Add *B* to *A* slowly, stirring until it cools to 35°C.

This is a smooth, white, free-flowing lotion of medium viscosity. It can be used alone as an emollient and protective agent or combined with therapeutic agents, e.g., benzyl benzoate.

LONGLOTION

		grams
A.	Cetyl Alcohol	2.600
	White Petrolatum	1.000
	White Beeswax	0.400
B.	Glycerin	1.600
	Sodium Lauryl Sulfate	0.200
	Distilled Water	94.200
	Methyl Paraben	0.015
	Propyl Paraben	0.015

Heat *A* to 70°C. Heat *B* to 70°C. on a water bath. Add *B* to *A* slowly, stirring until it cools to 35°C.

This is a smooth, light-bodied, nongreasy lotion of low viscosity. It spreads evenly over large areas and can be incorporated with a wide range of therapeutic agents, e.g., methyl salicylate.

POLOLOTION

		grams
A.	Stearic Acid	1.500
	Self-Emulsifying Glyceryl Monostearate	2.250

	White Petrolatum	5.250
	White Beeswax	1.000
B.	Sodium Lauryl Sulfate	0.150
	Glycerin	1.350
	Distilled Water	88.500
	Methyl Paraben	0.015
	Propyl Paraben	0.015

Heat *A* to 75°C. Heat *B* to 75°C. on a water bath. Add *B* to *A* slowly, stirring until it cools to 35°C.

This homogeneous, light-bodied lotion flows freely and spreads readily. It is useful for general-purpose work and combines with a large number of dermatological agents, such as bismuth subnitrate or vitamin A concentrate.

ADALOTION

		grams
A.	Cetyl Alcohol	2.750
	White Petrolatum	7.500
	White Beeswax	1.000
B.	Glycerin	1.500
	Sodium Lauryl Sulfate	0.250
	Distilled Water	87.000
	Methyl Paraben	0.015
	Propyl Paraben	0.015

Heat *A* to 75°C. Heat *B* to 75°C. on a water bath. Add *B* to *A* slowly, stirring until cooled to 35°C.

This smooth, light-bodied, free-flowing lotion can be used with many medicinal agents. Oily liquids and powdered drugs, such as olive oil, incorporate very easily and form good preparations.

LAUROLOTION

		grams
A.	Stearic Acid	5.650
	Cetyl Alcohol	1.650
B.	Sodium Lauryl Sulfate	0.350
	Glycerin	2.350
	Distilled Water	90.000

Methyl Paraben	0.015
Propyl Paraben	0.015

Heat *A* to 70°C. Heat *B* to 70°C. on a water bath. Add *B* to *A* slowly, stirring until it cools to 35°C.

This medium-bodied, homogeneous lotion is useful for general-purpose work. It is free-flowing, greaseless and easily removable with water. Precipitated sulfur is easily incorporated.

ERTHALOTION

		grams
A.	Stearyl Alcohol	1.000
	Self-Emulsifying Glyceryl Monostearate	1.850
	White Petrolatum	1.500
	Liquid Petrolatum	1.000
B.	Glycerin	1.650
	Distilled Water	93.000
	Methyl Paraben	0.015
	Propyl Paraben	0.015

Heat *A* to 70°C. Heat *B* to 70°C. on a water bath. Add *B* to *A* slowly, stirring until it cools to 35°C.

This nonionic, heavy-bodied, washable vehicle is suitable for use alone or with the majority of dermatological preparations. It flows easily and has good adhesive character. It yields a good lotion with solutions of sodium thiosulfate.

LODOLOTION

		grams
A.	Cetyl Alcohol	7.000
	White Petrolatum	7.250
	White Beeswax	0.130
B.	Glycerin	2.500
	Sodium Lauryl Sulfate	0.250
	Distilled Water	82.870
	Methyl Paraben	0.015
	Propyl Paraben	0.015

Heat *A* to 75°C. Heat *B* to 75°C. on a water bath. Add *A* to *B* slowly, stirring until it cools to 35°C.

This smooth, free-flowing lotion can be combined with many types of medication or used alone as an emollient and protective agent. It is particularly suitable for use with aqueous, alcoholic, and oily liquids.

MAYLOTION

		grams
A.	Stearyl Alcohol	4.600
	White Petrolatum	6.400
B.	Glycerin	2.000
	Sodium Lauryl Sulfate	0.200
	Distilled Water	86.800
	Methyl Paraben	0.015
	Propyl Paraben	0.015

Heat *A* to 75°C. Heat *B* to 75°C. on a water bath. Add *B* to *A* slowly, stirring until it cools to 35°C.

This medium-bodied preparation flows easily and can be removed readily with water. The majority of medicinal agents can be incorporated, such as methyl salicylate or Burow's solution.

PHARMLOTION

		grams
A.	Self-Emulsifying Glyceryl Monostearate	3,750
	White Petrolatum	5.000
	Liquid Petrolatum	0.750
	White Beeswax	0.500
B.	Glycerin	1.750
	Distilled Water	88.250
	Methyl Paraben	0.015
	Propyl Paraben	0.015

Heat *A* to 70°C. Heat *B* to 70°C. on a water bath. Add *B* to *A* slowly stirring until 35°C.

This smooth, medium-bodied, nonionic lotion combines with most therapeutic agents, such as lime water or castor oil.

WARALOTION

		grams
A.	Cetyl Alcohol	3.000

Liquid Petrolatum	8.000
White Beeswax	1.000
B. Sodium Lauryl Sulfate	1.000
Distilled Water	87.000
Methyl Paraben	0.015
Propyl Paraben	0.015

Heat *A* to 70°C. Heat *B* to 70°C. on a water bath. Add *B* to *A* slowly, stirring until it cools to 40°C.

This is a highly compatible, nongreasy, light-bodied lotion. It flows freely and can be easily applied to large areas. It is very useful as an emollient and absorbs powdered medications. Benzyl benzoate, pyrogallol, or calamine can be incorporated.

PROVALOTION

	grams
Stearic Acid	3.000
Cetyl Alcohol	0.400
Self-Emulsifying Glyceryl Monostearate	1.000
White Petrolatum	4.800
Span 60*	0.800
Tween 40*	0.400
Distilled Water	89.600
Methyl Paraben	0.015
Propyl Paraben	0.015

Heat all together to 80°C. on a water bath. Stir slowly until it cools to 35°C.

This is a smooth, medium-bodied, nonionic vehicle. It flows easily and is readily combined with all classes of medication, especially in the liquid state. Rose water or witch hazel can be incorporated very well.

*Atlas Powder Co.

SINDLOTION

	grams
A. Spermaceti	3.350
Cetyl Alcohol	2.350
White Petrolatum	0.650
White Beeswax	2.300

B.	Glycerin	2.000
	Sodium Lauryl Sulfate	0.350
	Distilled Water	89.000
	Methyl Paraben	0.015
	Propyl Paraben	0.015

Heat *A* to 70°C. Heat *B* to 70°C. on a water bath. Add *B* to *A* slowly, stirring until it cools to 35°C.

This medium-bodied, free-flowing lotion is quite greaseless. Light powders or liquids, such as tannic acid or iodohydroxy quinoline compounds, are compatible with this lotion.

PARTLOTION

		grams
A.	Stearic Acid	3.000
	Stearyl Alcohol	1.000
	White Petrolatum	5.000
	Liquid Petrolatum	2.500
	White Beeswax	1.000
B.	Sodium Lauryl Sulfate	0.250
	Distilled Water	87.250
	Methyl Paraben	0.015
	Propyl Paraben	0.015

Heat *A* to 75°C. Heat *B* to 75°C. on a water bath. Add *B* to *A* slowly, stirring until it cools to 35°C.

This smooth, light-bodied lotion spreads easily. It is comparatively greaseless and mixes well with a large number of therapeutic agents. Powdered drugs, such as zinc oxide or starch, are easy to incorporate.

SERRALOTION

		grams
A.	Cetyl Alcohol	3.750
	White Petrolatum	6.500
	White Beeswax	0.750
B.	Glycerin	1.750
	Sodium Lauryl Sulfate	0.250
	Distilled Water	87.000
	Methyl Paraben	0.015
	Propyl Paraben	0.015

Heat *A* to 70°C. Heat *B* to 70°C. on a water bath. Add *B* to *A* slowly, stirring until it cools to 35°C.

This homogeneous, medium-bodied preparation is suitable for general-purpose work. It blends well with aqueous and alcoholic liquids, such as boric acid solution, camphor water, or liquor carbonis detergens.

MAXILOTION

	grams
A. Stearyl Alcohol	4.750
White Petrolatum	4.750
White Beeswax	0.500
B. Glycerin	1.500
Sodium Lauryl Sulfate	0.250
Distilled Water	88.250
Methyl Paraben	0.015
Propyl Paraben	0.015

Heat *A* to 70°C. Heat *B* to 70°C. on a water bath. Add *B* to *A* slowly, stirring until it cools to 35°C.

This smooth, heavy-bodied, greaseless preparation flows easily, absorbs liquids readily, and is washable. It can be used for general-purpose work. Copper sulfate solution or sodium thiosulfate solution is easy to incorporate.

DELVILOTION

	grams
A. Spermaceti	7.500
Self-Emulsifying Glyceryl Monostearate	4.500
Span 60*	3.000
B. Tween 40*	2.000
Glycerin	3.000
Distilled Water	80.000
Methyl Paraben	0.015
Propyl Paraben	0.015

Heat *A* to 70°C. Heat *B* to 70°C. on a water bath. Add *B* to *A* slowly, stirring until it cools to 35°C.

This nonionic, light-bodied, greaseless, washable vehicle is compatible with all types of medication. It flows freely and can be easily applied to large areas. Oily liquids combine well with it and methyl salicylate or phenol are easy to incorporate.

---

*Atlas Powder Co.

TOPLOTION

		grams
A.	Stearyl Alcohol	1.000
	Self-Emulsifying Glyceryl Monostearate	2.500
	White Petrolatum	3.500
B.	Glycerin	1.000
	Distilled Water	92.000
	Methyl Paraben	0.015
	Propyl Paraben	0.015

Heat *A* to 70°C. Heat *B* to 70°C. on a water bath. Add *B* to *A* slowly, stirring until it cools to 35°C.

This greaseless, nonionic, heavy-bodied, adhesive lotion flows, spreads, and washes off easily. Liquid medications, such as Burow's solution or benzyl, benzoate, combine best with this vehicle.

PATALOTION

		grams
A.	Spermaceti	1.000
	Stearyl Alcohol	4.000
	Peanut Oil	24.000
B.	Liquid Sorbitol	2.000
	Sodium Lauryl Sulfate	1.000
	Distilled Water	68.000
	Methyl Paraben	0.015
	Propyl Paraben	0.015

Heat *A* to 70°C. Heat *B* to 70°C. on a water bath. Add *B* to *A* slowly, stirring until it cools to 40°C.

This smooth, medium-bodied lotion has better than average emollient action. It is excellent for general-purpose work and easy to remove. It is very well suited for use with powdered drugs, such as magnesium oxide, sulfur, or resorcin.

CREAMLOTION

		grams
A.	Cetyl Alcohol	5.000
	White Petrolatum	7.500
	White Beeswax	0.250
B.	Glycerin	2.000
	Sodium Lauryl Sulfate	0.250
	Distilled Water	85.000
	Methyl Paraben	0.015
	Propyl Paraben	0.015

Heat *A* to 75°C. Heat *B* to 75°C. on a water bath. Add *B* to *A* slowly, stirring until it cools to 40°C.

This smooth, heavy-bodied, adhesive lotion is suitable for use with a large volume of aqueous liquid medication or as an emollient. It spreads well and takes up camphor water or boric acid solution readily.

SEGUALOTION

		grams
A.	Stearic Acid	4.000
	Self-Emulsifying Glyceryl Monostearate	1.650
	Liquid Petrolatum	6.350
B.	Glycerin	1.650
	Sodium Lauryl Sulfate	0.350
	Distilled Water	86.000
	Methyl Paraben	0.015
	Propyl Paraben	0.015

Heat *A* to 75°C. Heat *B* to 75°C. on a water bath. Add *B* to *A* slowly, stirring until it cools to 35°C.

This homogeneous, light-bodied vehicle flows freely and is practically greaseless. It is well adapted for general-purpose use. Powdered and liquid medication, such as calamine or solution of coal tar, combines well with this lotion.

JORDALOTION

		grams
A.	Stearyl Alcohol	2.000

	Cetyl Alcohol	1.800
	White Beeswax	0.400
	Span 60*	1.800
B.	Tween 40*	1.000
	Distilled Water	93.000
	Methyl Paraben	0.015
	Propyl Paraben	0.015

Heat *A* to 85°C. Heat *B* to 85°C. on a water bath. Add *B* to *A* slowly, stirring until it cools to 35°C.

This smooth, nonionic heavy-bodied, absorptive lotion is best suited for use with liquids, such as olive oil or boric acid solution.

*Atlas Powder Co.

PORTOLOTION

		grams
A.	Cetyl Alcohol	1.800
	Stearyl Alcohol	1.000
	White Beeswax	0.400
	White Petrolatum	4.600
B.	Sodium Lauryl Sulfate	0.200
	Glycerin	1.000
	Distilled Water	91.000
	Methyl Paraben	0.015
	Propyl Paraben	0.015

Heat *A* to 70°C. Heat *B* to 70°C. on a water bath. Add *B* to *A* slowly, stirring until it cools to 35°C.

This medium-bodied lotion is suitable for general-purpose use, especially combined with aqueous drug solutions.

SARLOTION

		grams
A.	Self-Emulsifying Glyceryl Monostearate	2.750
	Cetyl Alcohol	1.250
	White Petrolatum	2.500
	White Beeswax	1.250
B.	Glycerin	1.500

Distilled Water	90.750
Methyl Paraben	0.015
Propyl Paraben	0.015

Heat *A* to 70°C. Heat *B* to 70°C. on a water bath. Add *B* to *A* slowly, stirring until it cools to 35°C.

This medium-bodied, greaseless, nonionic lotion can be used alone as an emollient or in combination with therapeutic agents, such as Burow's or coal-tar solutions.

PRACTOLOTION

		grams
A.	Spermaceti	3.000
	Cetyl Alcohol	2.000
	Liquid Petrolatum	20.000
B.	Sodium Lauryl Sulfate	1.000
	Proplyene Glycol	2.000
	Distilled Water	72.000
	Methyl Paraben	0.015
	Propyl Paraben	0.015

Heat *A* to 70°C. Heat *B* to 70°C. on a water bath. Add *B* to *A* slowly, stirring until it cools to 40°C.

This homogeneous, medium-bodied, washable vehicle is suitable for general-purpose use. It is compatible with both oily and aqueous agents. Copper sulfate solution or cod-liver oil can be incorporated.

COMPLOTION

		grams
A.	Stearic Acid	4.000
	Stearyl Alcohol	1.000
	White Petrolatum	2.250
	White Beeswax	1.250
B.	Propylene Glycol	1.250
	Sodium Lauryl Sulfate	0.250
	Distilled Water	90.000
	Methyl Paraben	0.015
	Propyl Paraben	0.015

Heat *A* to 75°C. Heat B to 75°C. on a water bath. Add *B* to *A* slowly, stirring until it cools to 35°C.

This light-bodied greaseless lotion flows easily and is suitable for application to large areas. Most types of medication, especially powders, can be combined with it. Calamine and sulfur yield a homogeneous mixture.

CENTRALOTION

		grams
A.	Cetyl Alcohol	3.600
	White Beeswax	0.400
B.	Glycerin	1.800
	Sodium Lauryl Sulfate	0.200
	Distilled Water	94.000
	Methyl Paraben	0.015
	Propyl Paraben	0.015

Heat *A* to 70°C. Heat *B* to 70°C. on a water bath. Add *B* to *A* slowly, stirring until it cools to 35°C.

This smooth, light, nongreasy lotion spreads freely over large areas. It can be used as an emollient or as a vehicle for medication, such as olive oil.

DELTILOTION

		grams
A.	Stearyl Alcohol	3.000
	White Petrolatum	6.250
	Liquid Petrolatum	1.250
	White Beeswax	1.000
B.	Glycerin	1.500
	Sodium Lauryl Sulfate	0.250
	Distilled Water	86.750
	Methyl Paraben	0.015
	Propyl Paraben	0.015

Heat *A* to 70°C. Heat *B* to 70°C. on a water bath. Add *B* to *A* slowly, stirring until it cools to 35°C.

This smooth, medium-bodied preparation can be used with a wide range of solid or liquid therapeutic agents. Resorcin or phenol combine very well to form a homogeneous lotion.

NORMALOTION

		grams
A.	Cetyl Alcohol	2.850
	Stearyl Alcohol	1.250
	White Petrolatum	3.750
B.	Glycerin	1.500
	Sodium Lauryl Sulfate	0.150
	Distilled Water	90.500
	Methyl Paraben	0.015
	Propyl Paraben	0.015

Heat *A* to 70°C. Heat *B* to 70°C. on a water bath. Add *B* to *A* slowly, stirring until it cools to 35°C.

This homogeneous, smooth-textured lotion of medium body can be applied easily to large areas. Most types of medication, especially oily liquids, are well incorporated into this lotion.

PETROLOTION

	grams
Self-Emulsifying Glyceryl Monostearate	4.650
White Petrolatum	7.000
Glycerin	1.350
Distilled Water	87.000
Methyl Paraben	0.015
Propyl Paraben	0.015

Heat all together to 70°C. on a water bath. Stir slowly until it cools to 35°C.

This smooth, nonionic heavy-bodied lotion is compatible with most medication. Liquids, e.g., camphor water or phenol solutions, are easily combined with this preparation.

KOMBALOTION

		grams
A.	Cetyl Alcohol	2.500

	Stearyl Alcohol	1.250
	White Petrolatum	8.250
	White Beeswax	1.000
B.	Glycerin	2.250
	Sodium Lauryl Sulfate	0.250
	Distilled Water	84.500
	Methyl Paraben	0.015
	Propyl Paraben	0.015

Heat *A* to 70°C. Heat *B* to 70°C. on a water bath. Add *B* to *A* slowly, stirring until it cools to 35°C.

This medium-bodied lotion is suitable for general-purpose use because most drugs are compatible with it. Oily liquids and essential oils, e.g., olive oil and oil of wintergreen, are taken up well.

AGRALOTION

		grams
A.	Spermaceti	2.500
	Cetyl Alcohol	1.000
	White Petrolatum	4.500
	Liquid Petrolatum	2.250
B.	Sodium Lauryl Sulfate	0.250
	Distilled Water	89.500
	Methyl Paraben	0.015
	Propyl Paraben	0.015

Heat *A* to 70°C. Heat *B* to 70°C. on a water bath. Add *B* to *A* slowly, stirring until it cools to 35°C.

This smooth, light-bodied, free-flowing, nongreasy lotion is satisfactory for use with powdered and liquid therapeutic agents. Benzocaine, lead subacetate and phenol are easily incorporated into this preparation.

TRULOTION

	grams
Self-Emulsifying Glyceryl Monostearate	4.250
White Petrolatum	8.250
Distilled Water	87.500
Methyl Paraben	0.015
Propyl Paraben	0.015

Heat all together to 65°C. on a water bath. Stir slowly until it cools to 35°C.

This nonionic, smooth, light-bodied lotion is suitable for application to large areas as an emollient or protective agent. Most drugs, such as benzocaine and tannic acid, can be used in combination with it.

TACTILOTION

		grams
A.	Cetyl Alcohol	4.000
	Stearyl Alcohol	3.350
	Liquid Petrolatum	4.800
	White Beeswax	2.000
B.	Sodium Lauryl Sulfate	0.350
	Distilled Water	85.500
	Methyl Paraben	0.015
	Propyl Paraben	0.015

Heat *A* to 70°C. Heat *B* to 70°C. on a water bath. Add *B* to *A* slowly, stirring until it cools to 35°C.

This light-bodied, free-flowing, washable lotion is suitable for use on large areas. It absorbs powdered medication. Starch, resorcin, and calamine are especially suitable.

DARLOTION

		grams
A.	Stearyl Alcohol	2.600
	White Petrolatum	2.000
	White Beeswax	0.400
B.	Propylene Glycol	1.000
	Sodium Lauryl Sulfate	0.200
	Distilled Water	93.800
	Methyl Paraben	0.015
	Propyl Paraben	0.015

Heat *A* to 70°C. Heat *B* to 70°C. on a water bath. Add *B* to *A* slowly, stirring until it cools to 40°C.

This homogeneous, heavy-bodied, washable lotion pours easily. It absorbs aqueous or alcoholic liquids, such as solutions of lead subacetate or lime water.

FLORALOTION

		grams
A.	Cetyl Alcohol	1.000
	Self-Emulsifying Glyceryl Monostearate	1.800
	White Petrolatum	1.000
	Liquid Petrolatum	3.000
B.	Glycerin	0.600
	Distilled Water	91.000
	Methyl Paraben	0.015
	Propyl Paraben	0.015

Heat *A* to 70°C. Heat *B* to 70°C. on a water bath. Add *B* to *A* slowly, stirring until it cools to 35°C.

This light-bodied lotion of low viscosity spreads easily and flows freely. It is suitable for use on large areas. Combined with powders, such as benzocaine, talc, or precipitated sulfur, it gives a smooth homogeneous mixture.

WILLOTION

		grams
A.	Stearic Acid	2.000
	Cetyl Alcohol	2.250
	White Petrolatum	5.000
	White Beeswax	0.500
B.	Propylene Glycol	1.250
	Sodium Lauryl Sulfate	0.250
	Distilled Water	88.750
	Methyl Paraben	0.015
	Propyl Paraben	0.015

Heat *A* to 75°C. Heat *B* to 75°C. on a water bath. Add *B* to *A* slowly, stirring until it cools to 35°C.

This light-bodied lotion of low viscosity flows freely. Easily applied and readily removed with water, it is a good vehicle for resorcin, liquor carbonis detergens, and other aqueous or oily liquids.

SHARLOTION

	grams
Self-Emulsifying Glyceryl Monostearate	4.250

White Petrolatum	4.000
Glycerin	2.000
Distilled Water	89.750
Methyl Paraben	0.015
Propyl Paraben	0.015

Heat all together to 70°C. on a water bath. Stir slowly until it cools to 35°C.

This smooth, free-flowing, nonionic lotion of medium viscosity can be employed in combination with a large number of medicinal substances, or alone as an emollient or protective. Liquor carbonis detergens and olive oil combine well with this lotion.

DALYLOTION

		grams
A.	Cetyl Alcohol	5.000
	White Petrolatum	4.250
B.	Sodium Lauryl Sulfate	0.250
	Glycerin	1.750
	Distilled Water	88.750
	Methyl Paraben	0.015
	Propyl Paraben	0.015

Heat *A* to 70°C. Heat *B* to 70°C. on a water bath. Add *B* to *A* slowly, stirring until it cools to 35°C.

This is a smooth, free-flowing greaseless lotion of low viscosity and pleasing appearance. It is suitable for general-purpose use alone or in combination with medication. It combines well with powdered substances, such as calamine.

LOCHLOTION

		grams
A.	Stearyl Alcohol	2.600
	White Petrolatum	5.600
	White Beeswax	0.200
B.	Propylene Glycol	1.400
	Sodium Lauryl Sulfate	0.200
	Distilled Water	90.000
	Methyl Paraben	0.015

Propyl Paraben	0.015

Heat A to 70°C. Heat *B* to 70°C. on a water bath. Add *B* to *A* slowly, stirring until it cools to 35°C.

This smooth, medium-bodied, nongreasy, white lotion flows freely and spreads evenly on large areas. It is compatible with most medication, e.g., tincture of benzoin.

VIVALOTION

	grams
A. Cetyl Alcohol	2.350
Self-Emulsifying Glyceryl Monostearate	2.350
White Petrolatum	9.000
B. Sodium Lauryl Sulfate	0.300
Distilled Water	86.000
Methyl Paraben	0.015
Propyl Paraben	0.015

Heat *A* to 70°C. Heat *B* to 70°C. on a water bath. Add *B* to *A* slowly, stirring until it cools to 35°C.

This medium-bodied preparation is useful for general-purpose work. It can be combined with most medication or used alone as an emollient and protective. Solutions of coal tar, phenol or sulfur can be easily incorporated.

CALMLOTION

	grams
A. Stearic Acid	2.250
Self-Emulsifying Glyceryl Monostearate	2.500
Liquid Petrolatum	2.000
White Beeswax	0.750
B. Glycerin	1.000
Distilled Water	91.500
Methyl Paraben	0.015
Propyl Paraben	0.015

Heat *A* to 75°C. Heat *B* to 75°C. on a water bath. Add *B* to *A* slowly, stirring until it cools to 35°C.

This greaseless, light-bodied nonionic lotion is free flowing and compatible with most dermatological agents. Methyl salicylate, benzocaine, and tannic acid combine very well with this lotion.

PYALOTION

		grams
A.	Liquid Petrolatum	12.000
	Stearyl Alcohol	4.000
B.	Glycerin	3.000
	Sodium Lauryl Sulfate	1.000
	Distilled Water	80.000
	Methyl Paraben	0.015
	Propyl Paraben	0.015

Heat *A* to 70°C. Heat *B* to 70°C. on a water bath. Add *B* to *A* slowly, stirring until it cools to 40°C.

This homogeneous lotion of medium body spreads evenly, flows readily, adheres well, and can be removed with water. Practically all classes of therapeutic agents can be incorporated. Eutectic mixtures, such as camphor and menthol, or powdered drugs, are compatible with it.

ELBALOTION

		grams
A.	Self-Emulsifying Glyceryl Monostearate	3.350
	Spermaceti	3.000
	White Petrolatum	3.350
	Liquid Petrolatum	1.300
B.	Glycerin	2.000
	Distilled Water	87.000
	Methyl Paraben	0.015
	Propyl Paraben	0.015

Heat *A* to 70°C. Heat *B* to 70°C. on a water bath. Add *B* to *A* slowly, stirring until it cools to 35°C.

This nonionic, light-bodied free-flowing, greaseless lotion is a good emollient and protective. Almost any type of medication, e.g., tincture of benzoin and precipitated sulfur, can be added.

SPECILOTION

	grams
A. Cetyl Alcohol	2.350
White Petrolatum	5.350
White Beeswax	1.450
B. Glycerin	1.000
Sodium Lauryl Sulfate	0.350
Distilled Water	89.500
Methyl Paraben	0.015
Propyl Paraben	0.015

Heat *A* to 70°C. Heat *B* to 70°C. on a water bath. Add *B* to *A* slowly, stirring until it cools to 35°C.

This smooth, ready-flowing, heavy-bodied, adhesive vehicle is best suited for use with aqueous or alcoholic liquids, such as rose water or boric acid solution.

SPYROLOTION

	grams
A. Self-Emulsifying Glyceryl Monostearate	5.000
White Petrolatum	4.600
B. Propylene Glycol	2.200
Sodium Lauryl Sulfate	0.200
Distilled Water	89.000
Methyl Paraben	0.015
Propyl Paraben	0.015

Heat *A* to 75°C. Heat *B* to 75°C. on a water bath. Add *B* to *A* slowly, stirring until it cools to 35°C.

This medium-free-flowing, greaseless vehicle is an effective general-purpose lotion. It can be used alone as a skin lubricant or with medication, such as menthol or phenol.

CHARILOTION

	grams
A. Stearyl Alcohol	2.000
Cetyl Alcohol	1.350
White Petrolatum	8.000

	White Beeswax	1.450
B.	Glycerin	1.350
	Sodium Lauryl Sulfate	0.350
	Distilled Water	85.500
	Methyl Paraben	0.015
	Propyl Paraben	0.015

Heat *A* to 70°C. Heat *B* to 70°C. on a water bath. Add *B* to *A* slowly, stirring until it cools to 35°C.

This smooth, heavy-bodied lotion takes up liquids, such as Burow's solution, sodium thiosulfate solution, or tinctures, easily.

PROTOLOTION

		grams
A.	Self-Emulsifying Glyceryl Monostearate	3.750
	Liquid Petrolatum	10.500
B.	Glycerin	1.000
	Distilled Water	84.750
	Methyl Paraben	0.015
	Propyl Paraben	0.015

Heat *A* to 70°C. Heat *B* to 70°C. on a water bath. Add *B* to *A* slowly, stirring until it cools to 35°C.

Almost all categories of medication are compatible with this smooth, medium-bodied nonionic lotion. It readily absorbs liquids, e.g., tincture of benzoin.

DETRILOTION

		grams
A.	Cetyl Alcohol	3.350
	Stearyl Alcohol	3.350
	Self-Emulsifying Glyceryl Monostearate	2.450
	Liquid Petrolatum	10.000
B.	Glycerin	2.000
	Sodium Lauryl Sulfate	0.350
	Distilled Water	78.500
	Methyl Paraben	0.015
	Propyl Paraben	0.015

Heat *A* to 75°C. Heat *B* to 75°C. on a water bath. Add *B* to *A* slowly, stirring until it cools to 35°C.

This smooth, light-bodied greaseless, good general-purpose lotion can also be used alone as an emollient and protective. Phenol or resorcinol is easy to incorporate.

ALLOLOTION

		grams
A.	Stearyl Alcohol	1.000
	Spermaceti	4.500
	Liquid Petrolatum	5.500
	White Beeswax	0.500
B.	Glycerin	1.500
	Sodium Lauryl Sulfate	0.250
	Distilled Water	86.750
	Methyl Paraben	0.015
	Propyl Paraben	0.015

Heat *A* to 70°C. Heat *B* to 70°C. on a water bath. Add *B* to *A* slowly, stirring until it cools to 35°C.

This homogeneous, light-bodied lotion is convenient for use on large areas. It absorbs powders and liquids alike.

CLARALOTION

		grams
A.	Cetyl Alcohol	3.000
	Polyethylene Glycol 4000*	3.600
	White Petrolatum	2.600
B.	Glycerin	1.800
	Sodium Lauryl Sulfate	0.200
	Distilled Water	88.500
	Methyl Paraben	0.015
	Propyl Paraben	0.015

Heat *A* to 75°C. Heat *B* to 75°C. on a water bath. Add *B* to *A* slowly, stirring until it cools to 40°C.

This smooth, heavy-bodied, adhesive lotion is relatively greaseless, flows easily, and is removed quickly with water. It is compatible with liquid dermatological agents, such as phenol and oleic acid.

*Carbide & Carbon Chemicals Co.

REYLOTION

		grams
A.	Stearic Acid	2.000
	Stearyl Alcohol	2.000
	White Petrolatum	2.000
	Liquid Petrolatum	1.000
	Beeswax	0.770
B.	Glycerin	0.980
	Sodium Lauryl Sulfate	0.250
	Distilled Water	91.000
	Methyl Paraben	0.015
	Propyl Paraben	0.015

Heat *A* to 75°C. Heat *B* to 75°C. on a water bath. Add *B* to *A* slowly, stirring until it cools to 35°C.

This heavy-bodied adhesive lotion absorbs liquids, e.g., camphor water or copper sulfate solution, readily.

PRENALOTION

		grams
A.	Spermaceti	2.800
	Cetyl Alcohol	2.400
	White Petrolatum	3.600
B.	Sodium Lauryl Sulfate	0.200
	Distilled Water	91.000
	Methyl Paraben	0.015
	Propyl Paraben	0.015

Heat *A* to 70°C. Heat *B* to 70°C. on a water bath. Add *B* to *A* slowly, stirring until it cools to 35°C.

This smooth, white lotion of medium body flows easily and rinses off readily. It can be used alone or in combination with dermatological agents, such as phenol and olive oil.

TRIMLOTION

		grams
A.	Self-Emulsifying Glyceryl Monostearate	2.500
	White Beeswax	1.000
	White Petrolatum	5.000
	Stearyl Alcohol	1.000
B.	Glycerin	0.500
	Distilled Water	90.000
	Methyl Paraben	0.015
	Propyl Paraben	0.015

Heat *A* to 70°C. Heat *B* to 70°C. on a water bath. Add *B* to *A* slowly, stirring until it cools to 35°C.

This smooth, medium-bodied, nonionic lotion is well adapted for general-purpose use. It is compatible with most medications. Aqueous, alcoholic, and oleagenous liquids, such as tinctures, can be added.

REGULOTION

		grams
A.	Cetyl Alcohol	2.800
	Stearyl Alcohol	0.800
	White Petrolatum	5.600
	White Beeswax	1.200
B.	Sodium Lauryl Sulfate	0.200
	Liquid Sorbitol	1.200
	Distilled Water	88.200
	Methyl Paraben	0.015
	Propyl Paraben	0.015

Heat *A* to 70°C. Heat *B* to 70°C. on a water bath. Add *B* to *A* slowly, stirring until it cools to 35°C.

This smooth, white, medium-bodied lotion will take up a wide range of medicaments, including liquids. This is a good vehicle for sulfur and salicylic acid.

CHAPTER FOUR

NONWASHABLE WATER-IN-OIL UNGUENT BASES

VERDIBASE

		grams
A.	Stearic Acid	3.000
	White Petrolatum	40.000
	Liquid Petrolatum	4.400
	Arlacel–C*	5.500
	Cholesterol	1.000
B.	Sodium Lauryl Sulfate	0.100
	Distilled Water	41.000
	Methyl Paraben	0.015
	Propyl Paraben	0.015

Heat *A* to 85°C. Heat *B* to 85°C. on a water bath. Add *B* to *A* slowly, stirring until congealed.

This fine, smooth-textured vehicle of medium body can retain all classes of liquid and powdered therapeutic agents, e.g., cod-liver oil or balsam of Peru.

---

*Atlas Powder Co.

BERABASE

		grams
A.	Spermaceti	6.000
	Liquid Petrolatum	5.000
	White Petrolatum	37.000
	Cholesterol	0.500

	Arlacel–C*	5.000
B.	Sodium Lauryl Sulfate	0.100
	Distilled Water	46.100
	Methyl Paraben	0.015
	Propyl Paraben	0.015

Heat *A* to 85°C. Heat *B* to 85°C. on a water bath. Add *B* to *A* slowly, stirring until congealed.

This homogeneous, medium-bodied base has good liquid absorptive and emollient properties. Most dermatological agents, e.g., tincture of benzoin or salicylic acid, combine well with it.

*Atlas Powder Co.

DACTOBASE

		grams
A.	White Petrolatum	23.000
	Stearyl Alcohol	3.000
	Liquid Petrolatum	6.000
	White Beeswax	4.000
	Arlacel–C*	6.000
B.	Distilled Water	58.000
	Methyl Paraben	0.015
	Propyl Paraben	0.015

Heat *A* to 70°C. Heat *B* to 70°C. on a water bath. Add *B* to *A* slowly, stirring until congealed.

This smooth, medium-bodied, nonionic vehicle is compatible with all classes of therapeutic agents. It can absorb several times its weight of aqueous liquids, but will not wash off with water. It can be used alone as an emollient and protective or with oily and aqueous liquids, such as methyl salicylate or boric acid solution.

*Atlas Powder Co.

SPONBASE

		grams
A.	Liquid Petrolatum	7.000
	White Petrolatum	34.000

	Cholesterol	2.000
	Span 60*	6.000
B.	Distilled Water	51.000
	Methyl Paraben	0.015
	Propyl Paraben	0.015

Heat *A* to 85°C. Heat *B* to 85°C. on a water bath. Add *B* to *A* slowly, stirring until congealed.

This nonionic, medium-bodied base absorbs powdered medication and large amounts of liquids. It takes up eutectic mixtures, e.g., lime water or camphor and menthol. It is a good emollient and lubricant when used alone.

*Atlas Powder Co.

DALBASE

		grams
A.	Stearic Acid	5.400
	White Petrolatum	34.000
	Liquid Petrolatum	7.000
	Arlacel–C*	5.000
B.	Sodium Lauryl Sulfate	0.100
	Distilled Water	48.500
	Methyl Paraben	0.015
	Propyl Paraben	0.015

Heat *A* to 75°C. Heat *B* to 75°C. on a water bath. Add *B* to *A* slowly, stirring until congealed.

This well-balanced absorptive vehicle of medium body is compatible with a wide range of medicinal agents. Oil of cade, or benzyl benzoate is easily incorporated to form a good unguent.

*Atlas Powder Co.

ENTROBASE

		grams
A.	Liquid Petrolatum	5.000
	White Petrolatum	41.000
	Arlacel–C*	6.000

B.	Sodium Lauryl Sulfate	0.100
	Distilled Water	47.900
	Methyl Paraben	0.015
	Propyl Paraben	0.015

Heat *A* to 70°C. Heat *B* to 70°C. on a water bath. Add *B* to *A* slowly, stirring until congealed.

This good emollient base of medium body spreads very evenly. Most liquid and powdered dermatological agents can be incorporated easily, such as precipitated sulfur or salicylic acid.

*Atlas Powder Co.

DIABASE

		grams
A.	Stearyl Alcohol	8.000
	White Petrolatum	39.000
	Arlacel–C*	6.900
B.	Sodium Lauryl Sulfate	0.100
	Distilled Water	46.000
	Methyl Paraben	0.015
	Propyl Paraben	0.015

Heat *A* to 75°C. Heat *B* to 75°C. on a water bath. Add *B* to *A* slowly, stirring until congealed.

This smooth, medium-bodied base is a good emollient and lubricant. It is compatible with all classes of medicinal agents and can absorb large volumes of liquids, such as calomel, ammoniated mercury or witch hazel.

*Atlas Powder Co.

TYROBASE

		grams
A.	White Petrolatum	37.000
	Self-Emulsifying Glyceryl Monostearate	2.500
	Liquid Petrolatum	5.000
	Arlacel–C*	5.500
	White Beeswax	1.000
B.	Sodium Lauryl Sulfate	0.100

Distilled Water	48.900
Methyl Paraben	0.015
Propyl Paraben	0.015

Heat *A* to 75°C. Heat *B* to 75°C. on a water bath. Add *B* to *A* slowly, stirring until congealed.

This preparation of medium body absorbs liquids readily and spreads easily. It is a good emollient and combines with a large number of medicinal agents, e.g., olive oil and calamine.

*Atlas Powder Co.

SILKBASE

		grams
A.	White Petrolatum	31.000
	Liquid Petrolatum	9.000
	White Beeswax	6.000
	Arlacel–C*	7.000
B.	Distilled Water	47.000
	Methyl Paraben	0.015
	Propyl Paraben	0.015

Heat *A* to 65°C. Heat *B* to 65°C. on a water bath. Add *B* to *A* slowly, stirring until congealed.

This nonionic, medium-bodied preparation spreads and adheres very well. It can be used alone as an emollient and lubricant or combined with various types of medication. It absorbs several times its weight of aqueous and other liquids and also powdered drugs.

*Atlas Powder Co.

CLERABASE

		grams
A.	Spermaceti	3.000
	White Petrolatum	39.000
	Liquid Petrolatum	4.000
	Arlacel–C*	4.500
B.	Sodium Lauryl Sulfate	0.100
	Distilled Water	49.400

Methyl Paraben	0.015
Propyl Paraben	0.015

Heat *A* to 70°C. Heat *B* to 70°C. on a water bath. Add *B* to *A* slowly, stirring until congealed.

This homogeneous, medium-bodied base is compatible with most powdered and liquid therapeutic agents, such as zinc oxide, boric acid, or methyl salicylate.

*Atlas Powder Co.

BODIBASE

		grams
A.	Liquid Petrolatum	3.000
	White Petrolatum	42.000
	Cholesterol	0.500
	Arlacel–C*	5.000
B.	Sodium Lauryl Sulfate	0.100
	Distilled Water	49.400
	Methyl Paraben	0.015
	Propyl Paraben	0.015

Heat *A* to 85°C. Heat *B* to 85°C. on a water bath. Add *B* to *A* slowly, stirring until congealed.

This smooth, medium-bodied vehicle has good liquid absorption and emollient properties. Liquid, semiliquid, and powdered therapeutic agents, such as tannic acid or phenol, can be combined with this lubricating, nonwashable base.

*Atlas Powder Co.

ESTABASE

		grams
A.	Stearyl Alcohol	1.500
	Cetyl Alcohol	3.000
	White Petrolatum	38.000
	Liquid Petrolatum	4.000
	White Beeswax	1.500
	Arlacel–C*	5.000

Arlacel–C*	5.000
B. Sodium Lauryl Sulfate	0.100
Distilled Water	50.000
Methyl Paraben	0.015
Propyl Paraben	0.015

Heat *A* to 85°C. Heat *B* to 85°C. on a water bath. Add *B* to *A* slowly, stirring until congealed.

This smooth, white preparation of medium body spreads easily and is compatible with a large number of dermatological agents, such as olive oil or ichthammol.

*Atlas Powder Co.

ABSORBASE

	grams
A. White Petrolatum	36.000
Arlacel–C*	6.000
White Beeswax	4.000
B. Distilled Water	54.000
Methyl Paraben	0.015
Propyl Paraben	0.015

Heat *A* to 65°C. Heat *B* to 65°C. on a water bath. Add *B* to *A* slowly, stirring until congealed.

This nonionic, medium-bodied vehicle absorbs powdered and liquid therapeutic agents, e.g., calamine, olive oil, and camphor water.

*Atlas Powder Co.

DEPABASE

	grams
A. Stearyl Alcohol	2.400
White Petrolatum	38.000
Liquid Petrolatum	6.000
Cholesterol	0.500
Arlacel–C*	6.000
B. Sodium Lauryl Sulfate	0.100
Distilled Water	47.000

Methyl Paraben	0.015
Propyl Paraben	0.015

Heat *A* to 85°C. Heat *B* to 85°C. on a water bath. Add *B* to *A* slowly, stirring until congealed.

This is a good, general-purpose base of medium body. It absorbs aqueous, oily, and alcoholic liquids as well as powdered medications, e.g., solutions of coal tar.

*Atlas Powder Co.

CHOLEBASE

		grams
A.	White Petrolatum	40.400
	Liquid Petrolatum	4.000
	Cholesterol	0.500
	Arlacel–C*	6.000
B.	Sodium Lauryl Sulfate	0.100
	Distilled Water	49.000
	Methyl Paraben	0.015
	Propyl Paraben	0.015

Heat *A* to 85°C. Heat *B* to 85°C. on a water bath. Add *B* to *A* slowly, stirring until congealed.

This fine-textured, homogeneous, absorbent vehicle of medium body has good emollient properties as a skin lubricant. It spreads evenly and is compatible with the majority of therapeutic agents, such as phenol.

*Atlas Powder Co.

RINOBASE

		grams
A.	Stearic Acid	2.000
	Stearyl Alcohol	7.000
	White Petrolatum	35.000
	Liquid Petrolatum	10.000
	Cholesterol	1.000
	Arlacel–C*	8.000

B.	Sodium Lauryl Sulfate	0.100
	Distilled Water	36.900
	Methyl Paraben	0.015
	Propyl Paraben	0.015

Heat *A* to 85°C. Heat *B* to 85°C. on a water bath. Add *B* to *A* slowly, stirring until congealed.

This good, homogeneous preparation of medium body spreads very easily. Liquid, semiliquid and powdered medicaments of all classes, such as benzyl benzoate or precipitated sulfur, can be incorporated.

*Atlas Powder Co.

ONTOBASE

		grams
A.	Cetyl Alcohol	9.000
	White Petrolatum	37.900
	White Beeswax	2.000
	Arlacel–C*	8.000
B.	Sodium Lauryl Sulfate	0.100
	Distilled Water	43.000
	Methyl Paraben	0.015
	Propyl Paraben	0.015

Heat *A* to 70°C. Heat *B* to 70°C. on a water bath. Add *B* to *A* slowly, stirring until congealed.

This smooth-textured, heavy-bodied base of good absorptive character retains all types of liquids and powders, such as camphor, menthol, and phenol.

*Atlas Powder Co.

INTOBASE

		grams
A.	Spermaceti	11.000
	Liquid Petrolatum	10.000
	White Beeswax	3.000
	White Petrolatum	24.000
	Cholesterol	1.000
	Arlacel–C*	6.000

B.	Sodium Lauryl Sulfate	0.100
	Distilled Water	44.900
	Methyl Parapen	0.015
	Propyl Paraben	0.015

Heat *A* to 85°C. Heat *B* to 85°C. on a water bath. Add *B* to *A* slowly, stirring until congealed.

This is a well-balanced, moderately oily vehicle of heavy body. It has good adhesive and liquid-absorption properties and is well adapted for use with medicinal agents of an oily nature, such as balsam of Peru and olive oil.

---

*Atlas Powder Co.

LATABASE

		grams
A.	Stearyl Alcohol	8.000
	Spermaceti	2.000
	White Petrolatum	35.000
	Arlacel–C*	6.900
B.	Sodium Lauryl Sulfate	0.100
	Distilled Water	48.000
	Methyl Paraben	0.015
	Propyl Paraben	0.015

Heat *A* to 70°C. Heat *B* to 70°C. on a water bath. Add *B* to *A* slowly, stirring until congealed.

This homogeneous, medium-bodied, liquid-absorbent vehicle is compatible with dermatological agents of all types, e.g., cod-liver oil or the concentrates of vitamins A and D.

---

*Atlas Powder Co.

OVABASE

		grams
A.	Cetyl Alcohol	7.000
	White Petrolatum	30.000
	White Beeswax	2.000
	Liquid Petrolatum	7.900
	Arlacel–C*	8.000

B. Sodium Lauryl Sulfate	0.100
Distilled Water	45.000
Methyl Paraben	0.015
Propyl Paraben	0.015

Heat *A* to 70°C. Heat *B* to 70°C. on a water bath. Add *B* to *A* slowly, stirring until congealed.

This smooth-textured, medium-bodied preparation spreads easily and absorbs liquids readily. It can be used alone as a skin lubricant or combined with medicaments, such as bismuth subgallate and members of the oxyquinoline group.

---

*Atlas Powder Co.

Chapter Five

NONWASHABLE WATER-IN-OIL LOTIONS

ZONALOTION

	grams
A. Stearyl Alcohol	0.500
Liquid Petrolatum	56.000
Arlacel–C*	4.000
B. Sodium Lauryl Sulfate	0.100
Distilled Water	39.400
Methyl Paraben	0.015
Propyl Paraben	0.015

Heat *A* to 70°C. Heat *B* to 70°C. on a water bath. Add *B* to *A* slowly, stirring until it cools to 35°C.

This smooth, homogeneous preparation of medium body spreads easily. Aqueous solutions are absorbed only up to 60%. It is compatible with all types of therapeutic agents, e.g., resorcinol.

*Atlas Powder Co.

SALTILOTION

	grams
A. Spermaceti	1.000
Cholesterol	1.000
Liquid Petrolatum	55.000
Arlacel–C*	4.900
B. Sodium Lauryl Sulfate	0.100

Distilled Water	38.000
Methyl Paraben	0.015
Propyl Paraben	0.015

Heat *A* to 85°C. Heat *B* to 85°C. on a water bath. Add *B* to *A* slowly, stirring until it cools to 35°C.

This heavy-bodied, easy-flowing, liquid-absorbent lotion is compatible with the majority of therapeutic agents. It is most suitable for use with coal tar solutions, phenol or tinctures.

*Atlas Powder Co.

NOVALOTION

		grams
A.	Self-Emulsifying Glyceryl Monostearate	0.500
	Cetyl Alcohol	1.000
	Liquid Petrolatum	62.000
	Arlacel–C*	5.000
B.	Sodium Lauryl Sulfate	0.100
	Distilled Water	31.400
	Methyl Paraben	0.015
	Propyl Paraben	0.015

Heat *A* to 70°C. Heat *B* to 70°C. on a water bath. Add *B* to *A* slowly, stirring until it cools to 35°C.

This light-bodied lotion has excellent liquid-absorbing properties. It spreads easily and combines with most types of dermatological agents, such as cod-liver oil and zinc oxide.

*Atlas Powder Co.

STEMLOTION

		grams
A.	Liquid Petrolatum	64.000
	Cholesterol	1.900
	Arlacel–C*	6.000
B.	Sodium Lauryl Sulfate	0.100
	Distilled Water	28.000
	Methyl Paraben	0.015
	Propyl Paraben	0.015

Heat *A* to 85°C. Heat *B* to 85°C. on a water bath. Add *B* to *A* slowly, stirring until it cools to 35°C.

This fine, light-bodied, free-flowing lotion may serve as a lubricant and protective agent or as a carrier for all types of medication. It absorbs liquids and combines with powders.

---

*Atlas Powder Co.

VERNALOTION

		grams
A.	Cetyl Alcohol	1.000
	Stearyl Alcohol	0.500
	Cholesterol	0.500
	Liquid Petrolatum	55.000
	Arlacel–C*	4.900
B.	Sodium Lauryl Sulfate	0.100
	Distilled Water	38.000
	Methyl Paraben	0.015
	Propyl Paraben	0.015

Heat *A* to 85°C. Heat *B* to 85°C. on a water bath. Add *B* to *A* slowly, stirring until it cools to 35°C.

This smooth, medium-bodied absorptive lotion, which is well suited for general-purpose use, is especially good for alcoholic liquids. It combines well with solutions of coal tar.

---

*Atlas Powder Co.

SADLOTION

		grams
A.	Self-Emulsifying Glyceryl Monostearate	1.000
	Spermaceti	1.500
	Liquid Petrolatum	59.000
	Arlacel–C*	5.000
B.	Sodium Lauryl Sulfate	0.100
	Distilled Water	33.400
	Methyl Paraben	0.015
	Propyl Paraben	0.015

Heat *A* to 70°C. Heat *B* to 70°C. on a water bath. Add *B* to *A* slowly, stirring until it cools to 35°C.

This light-bodied lotion is well adapted for general-purpose use. It can be employed as a vehicle for aqueous, oily or powdered medication, such as calamine or methyl salicylate.

*Atlas Powder Co.

CHERILOTION

		grams
A.	Cetyl Alcohol	1.500
	Cholesterol	0.500
	Liquid Petrolatum	53.000
	Arlacel–C*	3.900
B.	Sodium Lauryl Sulfate	0.100
	Distilled Water	41.000
	Methyl Paraben	0.015
	Propyl Paraben	0.015

Heat *A* to 85°C. Heat *B* to 85°C. on a water bath. Add *B* to *A* slowly, stirring until it cools to 35°C.

This smooth, medium-bodied absorptive vehicle can be combined with a large number of medicaments or used alone as an emollient. Phenol combines easily with this preparation.

*Atlas Powder Co.

PHAROLOTION

		grams
A.	Liquid Petrolatum	56.000
	Cholesterol	2.000
	Arlacel–C*	3.900
B.	Sodium Lauryl Sulfate	0.100
	Distilled Water	38.000
	Methyl Paraben	0.015
	Propyl Paraben	0.015

Heat *A* to 85°C. Heat *B* to 85°C. on a water bath. Add *B* to *A* slowly, stirring until it cools to 35°C.

This heavy-bodied, adhesive vehicle can be incorporated with a wide range of medicinal agents, e.g., alcoholic solutions of menthol or camphor.

*Atlas Powder Co.

APPLILOTION

		grams
A.	Cetyl Alcohol	0.500
	Stearyl Alcohol	0.500
	Liquid Petrolatum	54.000
	Arlacel–C*	3.900
B.	Sodium Lauryl Sulfate	0.100
	Distilled Water	41.000
	Methyl Paraben	0.015
	Propyl Paraben	0.015

Heat *A* to 70°C. Heat *B* to 70°C. on a water bath. Add *B* to *A* slowly, stirring until it cools to 35°C.

This medium-bodied liquid-absorptive lotion combines well with medicinal agents, such as β-naphthol or boric acid. Alone, it is a good lubricant.

*Atlas Powder Co.

NIROLOTION

		grams
A.	Self-Emulsifying Glyceryl Monostearate	1.000
	Stearic Acid	1.000
	Liquid Petrolatum	46.000
	Arlacel–C*	4.900
B.	Sodium Lauryl Sulfate	0.100
	Distilled Water	47.000
	Methyl Paraben	0.015
	Propyl Paraben	0.015

Heat *A* to 70°C. Heat *B* to 70°C. on a water bath. Add *B* to *A* slowly, stirring until it cools to 35°C.

This heavy-bodied vehicle absorbs only a moderate amount of

water. It can be combined with almost any medicinal agent, but is best with benzyl benzoate.

---

*Atlas Powder Co.

DELTALOTION

		grams
A.	Stearic Acid	0.500
	Cholesterol	1.000
	Liquid Petrolatum	45.000
	Arlacel–C*	4.000
B.	Sodium Lauryl Sulfate	0.100
	Distilled Water	49.400
	Methyl Paraben	0.015
	Propyl Paraben	0.015

Heat *A* to 85°C. Heat *B* to 85°C. on a water bath. Add *B* to *A* slowly, stirring until it cools to 35°C.

Most medicinal agents, e.g., methyl salicylate, are compatible with this medium-bodied vehicle. At first, it will absorb only half its weight of water. Additional small amounts can be added subsequently.

---

*Atlas Powder Co.

KENILOTION

		grams
A.	Cetyl Alcohol	3.000
	Liquid Petrolatum	52.000
	Arlacel–C*	4.900
B.	Sodium Lauryl Sulfate	0.100
	Distilled Water	40.000
	Methyl Paraben	0.015
	Propyl Paraben	0.015

Heat *A* to 70°C. Heat *B* to 70°C. on a water bath. Add *B* to *A* slowly, stirring until it cools to 35°C.

This smooth, preparation of medium body and good liquid absorption is compatible with the majority of medicinal agents, e.g., witch hazel.

---

*Atlas Powder Co.

MIRALOTION

	grams
A. Cetyl Alcohol	1.000
Stearic Acid	0.500
Liquid Petrolatum	57.000
Arlacel–C*	5.000
B. Sodium Lauryl Sulfate	0.100
Distilled Water	36.400
Methyl Paraben	0.015
Propyl Paraben	0.015

Heat *A* to 70°C. Heat *B* to 70°C. on a water bath. Add *B* to *A* slowly, stirring until it cools to 35°C.

This homogeneous, medium-bodied lotion combines with a wide range of medication. It is an especially good vehicle for sulfathiazole.

*Atlas Powder Co.

SIMLOTION

	grams
A. Stearyl Alcohol	1.500
Cetyl Alcohol	1.000
Liquid Petrolatum	48.000
Arlacel–C*	6.000
B. Sodium Lauryl Sulfate	0.100
Distilled Water	43.400
Methyl Paraben	0.015
Propyl Paraben	0.015

Heat *A* to 70°C. Heat *B* to 70°C. on a water bath. Add *B* to *A* slowly, stirring until it cools to 35°C.

This smooth, easy-flowing, heavy-bodied, absorptive lotion can be used as a simple emollient or protective. Many drugs are compatible with this lotion, but it is most useful with liquids, such as benzyl benzoate or methyl salicylate.

*Atlas Powder Co.

OLILOTION

	grams
A. Stearic Acid	2.000
Liquid Petrolatum	52.000
Arlacel–C*	3.900
B. Sodium Lauryl Sulfate	0.100
Distilled Water	41.000
Methyl Paraben	0.015
Propyl Paraben	0.015

Heat *A* to 70°C. Heat *B* to 70°C. on a water bath. Add *B* to *A* slowly, stirring until it cools to 35°C.

This smooth, heavy-bodied vehicle is compatible with most medicaments. It is adapted for combination with Burow's solution or coal tar solution.

*Atlas Powder Co.

OPRALOTION

	grams
A. Self-Emulsifying Glyceryl Monostearate	2.000
Liquid Petrolatum	54.000
Arlacel–C*	3.900
B. Sodium Lauryl Sulfate	0.100
Distilled Water	40.000
Methyl Paraben	0.015
Propyl Paraben	0.015

Heat *A* to 70°C. Heat *B* to 70°C. on a water bath. Add *B* to *A* slowly, stirring until it cools to 35°C.

This smooth, medium-bodied liquid-absorbent lotion combines with many therapeutic agents, such as tannic acid or aluminium chloride solution.

*Atlas Powder Co.

LIQUALOTION

	grams
A. Stearyl Alcohol	1.000

Spermaceti	1.500
Liquid Petrolatum	59.000
Arlacel–C*	6.000
B. Sodium Lauryl Sulfate	0.100
Distilled Water	32.400
Methyl Paraben	0.015
Propyl Paraben	0.015

Heat *A* to 70°C. Heat *B* to 70°C. on a water bath. Add *B* to *A* slowly, stirring until it cools to 35°C.

This light-bodied, nonionic, absorbent lotion can be combined with practically all dermatological agents. Aqueous, oily, and powdered medication can readily be incorporated.

*Atlas Powder Co.

HOSPILOTION

	grams
A. Liquid Petrolatum	60.000
Arlacel–C*	3.900
B. Sodium Lauryl Sulfate	0.100
Distilled Water	36.000
Methyl Paraben	0.015
Propyl Paraben	0.015

Heat *A* to 70°C. Heat *B* to 70°C. on a water bath. Add *B* to *A* slowly, stirring until it cools to 35°C.

This light-bodied, free-flowing vehicle is compatible with a wide variety of dermatological agents. Powdered drugs are very easily incorporated.

*Atlas Powder Co.

WITHLOTION

	grams
A. Stearyl Alcohol	1.000
Self-Emulsifying Glyceryl Monostearate	0.500
Cetyl Alcohol	0.500
Liquid Petrolatum	57.000
Arlacel–C*	4.900

B. Sodium Lauryl Sulfate	0.100
Distilled Water	36.000
Methyl Paraben	0.015
Propyl Paraben	0.015

Heat *A* to 70°C. Heat *B* to 70°C. on a water bath. Add *B* to *A* slowly, stirring until it cools to 35°C.

This medium-bodied liquid-absorbent lotion flows easily and spreads readily. It can be combined with most therapeutic agents, e.g., Burow's solution, or used alone as a lubricant and protective.

---

*Atlas Powder Co.

Chapter Six

OIL-IN-WATER WASHABLE ANHYDROUS UNGUENT BASES

KETABASE

	grams
Spermaceti	16
Tween 85*	10
Liquid Petrolatum	18
Polyethylene Glycol 1500†	39
Methyl Cellulose 1500‡	17

Heat all together to 72°C. on a water bath. Stir constantly until congealed.

This good, heavy-bodied, anhydrous base is suitable for general-purpose work. It can be employed with a wide range of dermatological agents where the absence of water is indicated or where aqueous liquids have a tendency to interfere with the therapeutic activity of medicaments. Camphor and menthol can be incorporated readily.

*Atlas Powder Co.
†Carbide & Carbon Chemicals Co.
‡Dow Chemical Co.

WUNBASE

	grams
Stearyl Alcohol	10
Spermaceti	9
White Petrolatum	5
Liquid Petrolatum	14

Polyethylene Glycol 1500*	44
Tween 85†	4
Methyl Cellulose 1500‡	14

Heat all together to 72°C. on a water bath. Stir constantly until congealed.

This heavy-bodied versatile anhydrous vehicle is compatible with dry or aqueous, oleaginous or alcoholic medicaments. β-Naphthol is an example.

*Carbide & Carbon Chemicals Co.
†Atlas Powder Co.
‡Dow Chemical Co.

SERENBASE

	grams
Cetyl Alcohol	19
Liquid Petrolatum	20
Tween 85*	9
Polyethylene Glycol 1500†	39
Methyl Cellulose 1500‡	13

Heat all together to 72°C. on a water bath. Stir constantly until congealed.

This well-balanced, nonionic heavy-bodied vehicle absorbs aqueous liquids and combines with most dermatological agents. It will not hydrolyze sensitive drugs. Resorcinol or menthol is very suitable for use with this vehicle.

*Atlas Powder Co.
†Carbide & Carbon Chemicals Co.
‡Dow Chemical Co.

FAIRBASE

	grams
Stearyl Alcohol	15
Stearic Acid	5
White Petrolatum	4
Liquid Petrolatum	15
Tween 85*	6
Polyethylene Glycol 1500†	40
Methyl Cellulose 1500‡	15

B.	Sodium Lauryl Sulfate	0.100
	Distilled Water	46.900
	Methyl Paraben	0.015
	Propyl Paraben	0.015

Heat *A* to 75°C. Heat *B* to 75°C. on a water bath. Add *B* to *A* slowly, stirring until congealed.

This medium-bodied vehicle is compatible with a wide range of medicaments. It is especially well adapted for use with crude coal tar and essential oils.

*Atlas Powder Co.

BEEBASE

		grams
A.	White Petrolatum	39.000
	Cetyl Aocohol	3.000
	Liquid Petrolatum	5.000
	White Beeswax	1.000
	Arlacel–C*	4.500
B.	Sodium Lauryl Sulfate	0.100
	Distilled Water	47.400
	Methyl Paraben	0.015
	Propyl Paraben	0.015

Heat *A* to 75°C. Heat *B* to 75°C. on a water bath. Add *B* to *A* slowly, stirring until congealed.

This is a good, medium-bodied, liquid-absorbing preparation which is oily but not greasy. It spreads easily and imparts a pleasant feeling to the skin surface. Most drugs are readily incorporated. Menthol, camphor or methyl salicylate combine very well with this vehicle.

*Atlas Powder Co.

GARDOBASE

		grams
A.	Self-Emulsifying Glyceryl Monostearate	1.000
	Liquid Petrolatum	4.400
	White Petrolatum	39.000
	Cholesterol	0.500

Heat all together to 72°C. on a water bath. Stir constantly until congealed.

This smooth absorbent preparation of heavy body can be spread and removed readily. It is good where the presence of aqueous liquids is detrimental to the compatibility or stability of the desired medication. However, water and water solutions can readily be incorporated. Calomel forms a fine unguent with this base.

---

*Atlas Powder Co.
†Carbide & Carbon Chemicals Co.
‡Dow Chemical Co.

PLIABASE

	grams
Stearic Acid	15
Self-Emulsifying Glyceryl Monostearate	10
Liquid Petrolatum	20
Polyethylene Glycol 1500*	37
Methyl Cellulose 1500†	18

Heat all together to 72°C. on a water bath. Stir constantly until congealed.

This absorbent, smooth base of heavy body can be combined with most aqueous, oily, or powdered therapeutic agents.

---

*Carbide & Carbon Chemicals Co.
†Dow Chemical Co.

EDELBASE

	grams
Cetyl Alcohol	10
Stearyl Alcohol	7
Liquid Petrolatum	17
Tween 85*	10
Polyethylene Glycol 1500†	38
Methyl Cellulose 1500‡	18

Heat all together to 72°C. on a water bath. Stir constantly until congealed.

This heavy-bodied preparation is compatible with most medications.

*Atlas Powder Co.
†Carbide & Carbon Chemicals Co.
‡Dow Chemical Co.

RETOBASE

	grams
Self-Emulsifying Glyceryl Monostearate	25
Liquid Petrolatum	18
Polyethylene Glycol 1500*	38
Methyl Cellulose 1500†	19

Heat all together to 72°C. on a water bath. Stir constantly until congealed.

This heavy-bodied, absorbent vehicle can be combined with a large number of liquid or powdered therapeutic agents, such as methyl salicylate.

*Carbide & Carbon Chemicals Co.
†Dow Chemical Co.

UNGUABASE

	grams
White Petrolatum	9
Self-Emulsifying Glyceryl Monostearate	20
Liquid Petrolatum	11
Polyethylene Glycol 1500*	34
Tween 85†	10
Methyl Cellulose 1500‡	16

Heat all together to 72°C. on a water bath. Stir constantly until congealed.

This smooth, heavy-bodied, water-absorbent preparation is compatible with a large number of dermatological agents, e.g., salicylic and benzoic acids.

*Carbide & Carbon Chemicals Co.
†Atlas Powder Co.
‡Dow Chemical Co.

DESORBASE

	grams
Stearic Acid	19
White Petrolatum	6
Liquid Petrolatum	12
Polyethylene Glycol 1500*	36
Tween 85†	10
Methyl Cellulose 1500‡	17

Heat all together to 72°C. on a water bath. Stir constantly until congealed.

This smooth, heavy-bodied, washable base can be combined with a large number of powdered and liquid therapeutic agents, such as balsam of Peru or solutions of coal tar. Medicinal agents that are sensitive to water can be incorporated with safety.

*Carbide & Carbon Chemicals Co.
†Atlas Powder Co.
‡Dow Chemical Co.

SEMABASE

	grams
Cetyl Alcohol	12
Spermaceti	7
White Petrolatum	4
Liquid Petrolatum	14
Tween 85*	10
Polyethylene Glycol 1500†	41
Methyl Cellulose 1500‡	12

Heat all together to 72°C. on a water bath. Stir constantly until congealed.

This smooth, heavy-bodied, absorptive base is compatible with all types of medicinal agents, such as Euresol or benzyl benzoate.

*Atlas Powder Co.
†Carbide & Carbon Chemicals Co.
‡Dow Chemical Co.

GRETABASE

	grams
Self-Emulsifying Glyceryl Monostearate	24
White Petrolatum	8
Liquid Petrolatum	13
Polyethylene Glycol 1500*	38
Tween 85†	8
Methyl Cellulose 1500‡	9

Heat all together to 72°C. on a water bath. Stir constantly until congealed.

This heavy-bodied vehicle can be combined directly with a wide range of powdered or liquid medicaments, e.g., ichthammol and phenol.

*Carbide & Carbon Chemicals Co.
†Atlas Powder Co.
‡Dow Chemical Co.

Chapter Seven

WATER-IN-OIL NONWASHABLE ANHYDROUS UNGUENT BASES

FORTABASE

	grams
Cetyl Alcohol	7
White Petrolatum	27
Liquid Petrolatum	9
White Beeswax	3
Arlacel–C*	9

Heat all together to 75°C. on a water bath. Stir slowly until congealed.

This is a medium-bodied, emollient absorption base. With olive oil it forms a fine, smooth-textured unguent.

*Atlas Powder Co.

VITRABASE

	grams
Spermaceti	10
White Petrolatum	70
Liquid Petrolatum	9
Cholesterol	1
Arlacel–C*	10

Heat all together to 85°C. on a water bath. Stir slowly until congealed.

This is a good general-purpose absorption base of medium body. It can retain several times its weight of water and is compatible with liquid and powdered therapeutic agents, such as methyl salicylate.

---

*Atlas Powder Co.

QUALIBASE

	grams
White Petrolatum	80
Liquid Petrolatum	10
Arlacel–C*	10

Heat all together to 70°C. on a water bath. Stir slowly until congealed.

This soft-bodied vehicle can take up large volumes of water. Practically all classes of medicinal agents can be easily incorporated, including powdered drugs.

---

*Atlas Powder Co.

PHYSIBASE

	grams
Self-Emulsifying Glyceryl Monostearate	5
White Petrolatum	74
Liquid Petrolatum	10
White Beeswax	2
Arlacel–C*	9

Heat all together to 75°C. on a water bath. Stir slowly until congealed.

This nonionic absorption base of medium body is capable of retaining several times its weight of water. It is compatible with most dermatological agents, e.g., crude coal tar.

---

*Atlas Powder Co., Wilmington, Del.

BONABASE

	grams
Stearic Acid	7

White Petrolatum	73
Liquid Petrolatum	8
Cholesterol	1
Arlacel–C*	11

Heat all together to 85°C. on a water bath. Stir slowly until congealed.

This homogeneous absorption base of medium body retains aqueous, oleaginous, and alcoholic liquids equally well. Powdered drugs, such as starch or calamine, can also be incorporated.

*Atlas Powder Co.

TOTABASE

	grams
Spermaceti	6
Liquid Petrolatum	8
White Petrolatum	77
Arlacel–C*	9

Heat all together to 70°C. on a water bath. Stir slowly until congealed.

This well-balanced preparation of medium body has the ability to absorb a considerable volume of liquid. Alone, it is an oily emollient and protective. It combines also with many drugs, such as castor oil or Burow's solution.

*Atlas Powder Co.

PARBASE

	grams
Stearyl Alcohol	2
Liquid Petrolatum	12
White Petrolatum	73
Cholesterol	1
Arlacel–C*	12

Heat all together to 85°C. on a water bath. Stir slowly until congealed.

This is a smooth, medium-bodied absorption base. Liquid medicaments and water-sensitive drugs are well suited for incorporation.

*Atlas Powder Co.

CREDOBASE

	grams
Cetyl Alcohol	6
Stearyl Alcohol	3
White Petrolatum	74
Liquid Petrolatum	7
Arlacel–C*	7
White Beeswax	3

Heat all together to 70°C. on a water bath. Stir slowly until congealed.

This smooth homogeneous base retains large amounts of liquid medicaments, e.g., cod-liver oil.

*Atlas Powder Co.

STUDABASE

	grams
Self-Emulsifying Glyceryl Monostearate	2
White Petrolatum	78
Liquid Petrolatum	9
Cholesterol	1
Arlacel–C*	10

Heat all together to 85°C. on a water bath. Stir slowly until congealed.

This is a very smooth, nonionic absorption base of medium body. It is compatible with the majority of dermatological agents, such as menthol and camphor.

*Atlas Powder Co.

ANABASE

	grams
White Petrolatum	79
Liquid Petrolatum	9

Cholesterol	1
Arlacel–C*	11

Heat all together to 85°C. on a water bath. Stir slowly until congealed.

This fine, smooth absorption base of medium body can be employed for general-purpose work or alone as an emollient and protective. It is especially recommended for use with water-sensitive drugs or with liquids, such as benzyl benzoate or copper sulfate solution.

*Atlas Powder Co.

ACTIBASE

	grams
Stearic Acid	9
Liquid Petrolatum	15
White Petrolatum	67
Arlacel–C*	9

Heat all together to 75°C. on a water bath. Stir slowly until congealed.

This very smooth, absorptive, nonionic vehicle of medium body is compatible with most medicaments in powdered or liquid form, e.g., zinc oxide or witch hazel.

*Atlas Powder Co.

SITUBASE

	grams
White Petrolatum	83
Liquid Petrolatum	6
Cholesterol	1
Arlacel–C*	10

Heat all together to 85°C. on a water bath. Stir slowly until congealed.

This medium-bodied, absorptive, nonionic vehicle can retain several times its weight of water. It is compatible with almost all medicaments, such as salicylic acid or rose water.

*Atlas Powder Co.

Bibliography

Assouly, M., *Arch. maladies profess.*, **7**:150 (1946).

Atkins, F., *Mfg. Chem.*, **21**:51 (1950).

Bamber, G., *Brit. J. Dermat.*, **52**:21 (1940).

Bandelin, F. J. and C. R. Kemp, *J. Am. Pharm. Assoc., Sci. Ed.*, **35**:66 (1946).

Barr, M., *Mid Atlantic Pharm.*, **1**:37 (1952).

Beeler, E., J.Am. Pharm.Assoc., *Pract. Pharm. Ed.*, **3**:231 (1942).

Boehm E., R. Williams, *Quart. J. Pharm.*, **16**:232 (1943).

Bennett, H., Practical Emulsions, New York, Chemical Publishing Co. (1943).

Berger, F., *Drogistenpraxis*, Berlin (1949).

Bergner, K. G., *Pharmazeutisches Taschenbuch*, Vienna (1938).

Berkman, S., and G. Egloff, *Emulsions and Foams*, New York, Reinhold Publishing Corp. (1941).

Berry, H., *Brit. Med. Bull.*, **3**:182 (1945).

Blok, C. J., *Opthalmologica*, **106**:57 (1943).

Bond, G. C., R. E. Hymanlech, and L. H. MacDonald, *J.Am.Pharm. Assoc., Pract. Pharm. Ed.*, **38**:30 (1949).

British Pharmacopoeia (1948).

Bruce, S., *Mfg. Chem.*, **21**:159 (1950).

Burrin, P. L., *J.Am.Pharm.Assoc., Pract.Pharm.Ed.*, **15**:32 (1954).

Burrows, A., and B. Russell, *Brit.Med.J.*, **2**:198 (1945).

Carbide and Carbon Chemical Co., *Emulsions and Detergents* (1949).

Catline, E. L., N. B. Cook, and S. F. Jeffries, *J.Am.Pharm.Assoc., Pract.Pharm.Ed.*, **11**:36 (1950).

Chamings, A.R.G., *Brit.J.Dermat.*, **58**:1 (1946).

Chilson, F., *Modern Cosmetics*, 2nd Ed., New York Drug and Cosmetic Industry.

Clayton, W., *Theory of Emulsions*, 3rd Ed., London, Churchill (1943).

Codex Medicamentarius Gallicus (1947).

Cook, E. F., and LaWall, *Remingtons Practice of Pharmacv*, 10th Ed., Easton, Pa., Mack Pub. Co. (1951).

Cox, C. L., and P. Goodrich, *J.Am.Pharm.Assoc., Pract. Pharm.Ed.*, **1**:210 (1940).
Crossen, G. E., *Pharmaceutical Preparations*, 3rd Ed., Philadelphia, Pa., Lea & Febiger (1952).
Dansk Farmaceutforening (1946).
DeNavarre, M. G., *The Chemistry and Manufacture of Cosmetics*, New York, D. Van Nostrand (1941).
Dorvault, F.L.M., *L'Officine Repertoire de Pharmacie*, 18th Ed., Paris (1945).
Draize, J. H., G. Woodart, and H. O. Calvary, *J.Pharmacol.Exptl. Ther.*, **82**:377 (1944).
Durvelle, J.P., *Preparation of Perfumes and Cosmetics*, London, Scott, Greenwood (1923).
Ehrenstein, E., *Am.Prof.Pharm.*, **16**:874 (1950).
Ellerbrock, A., *Arch.Dermatol.Syphilol.*, **191**:642 (1950).
Fiero, G. W., and A. Loomis, *J.Am.Pharm.Assoc., Scientific Ed.*, **34**:218 (1945).
Fiero, G. W., *Condensed Review of Pharmacy*, 7th Ed., New York, John Wiley (1952).
Fiero, G.W., *J.Am.Pharm.Assoc., Sci. Ed.*, **30**:145 (1941).
Fiero, G.W., *J.Am.Pharm.Assoc., Sci. Ed.*, **29**:502 (1940).
Fiero, G.W., and J. Dutcher, *J.Am.Pharm.Assoc., Sci.Ed.*, **34**:56 (1945).
Formulary, Bellvue Hospital (1948).
Formulary, New York Hospital (1951).
Formulary, University Hospital, Ann Arbor, Mich.,(1940).
Fowley, E., and C. O. Lee, *J.Am.Pharm.Assoc., Sci.Ed.*, **31**:105 (1942)
French, E. D., *Southern Med. J.*, **34**:284 (1941).
Gershenfeld, L., and A. Brilliant, *Am. J. Pharm.*, **111**:430 (1939).
Gershenfeld, L., *Am. J. Pharm.*, **112**:281 (1940).
Gershenfeld, L., and R. E. Miller, *Am. J. Pharm.*, **105**:194 (1933).
Gibson, H. A., H. E. Parker, and A. Almus, *J. Am. Pharm. Assoc., Sci. Ed.*, **30**:196 (1941).
Goldsmith, W. N., *Med. Press and Circ.*, **207**:294 (1942).
Goldsmith, W. N., *Brit. J. Dermatol.*, **52**:615 (1940).
Goldsmith, W. N., *Practitioner*, **156**:358 (1946).
Goldsmith, W. N., and F. F. Hillier, *Recent Advances in Dermatology*, New York, Blakiston (1954).
Goldstein, S. W., *J. Am. Pharm. Assoc., Pract. Pharm. Ed.*, **14**:111 (1953).
Goldstein, S. W., *J. Am. Pharm. Assoc., Pract. Pharm. Ed.*, **14**:710 (1953).
Goldstein, S. W., *J. Am. Pharm. Assoc., Pract. Pharm. Ed.*, **15**:41 (1954).

Goodman, W., *J. Am. Pharm. Assoc., Pract. Pharm. Ed.*, **3**:240 (1942).

Goodman, H., *Cosmetic Dermatology*, New York, McGraw-Hill (1936).

Goodman. H., *Dermatological Formulae*, Fort Pierce Beach, Fla., Forben Press, Inc. (1946).

Goodman, H., *Am. Profess. Pharmacist*, **8**:355 (1942).

Goodman, H., *Arch. Dermatol. Syphilol.*, **36**:116 (1936).

Greenberg, L. A., and D. Lester, *Handbook of Cosmetic Materials*, New York, Interscience (1954).

Gstirner, F., *Einführung in die Arzneibereitung*, Stuttgart (1949).

Hadengue, F., A. Radzievsky, and J. deLaneuvais, *Arch. maladies profess.*, **10**:257 (1949).

Hadgraft, J. W., and R. T. Brain, *Lancet*, **2**:78 (1949).

Hadgraft, J. W., *Pharm. J.*, **159**:222 (1947).

Hadgraft, J. W., and I. S. Bissett, *Pharm. J.*, **167**:66 (1951).

Hager, H., *Tratado de Farmacia*, Barcelona (1942).

Halpern, A., R. Muhich, and G. Siconolfi, *J. Am. Pharm. Assoc., Sci. Ed.*, **40**:6 (1951).

Harry, R. G., *Cosmetic Materials*, London, L. Hill, (1948).

Harry, R. G., *Brit. J. Dermatol.*, **53**:65 (1941).

Harry, R. G., *Modern Cosmeticology, 3rd Ed.*, New York, Chemical Publishing Co. (1947).

Hoffman, I. K., *J. Am. Pharm. Assoc., Pract. Pharm. Ed.*, **12**:475 (1951).

Holland, M. O., *Pharm. Internat.*, **6**:30 (1952).

Hopf., G., *Arch. Dermatol. u. Syphilis*, **181**:204 (1940).

Husa, W. J., *Pharmaceutical Dispensing, 3rd Ed.* (1947).

Huston, M. J., B. E. Riedel, J. R. Murray, and G. A. Groves, *Am. Profess. Pharmacist*, **15**:145 (1949).

Huyck, C. L., *Am. Profess. Pharmacist*, **15**:633 (1949).

Ice, C., and L. E. Harris, *J. Am. Pharm. Assoc.*, Sci. Ed., **32**:111 (1943).

Index Medicamentorum, Oslo (1945).

Anonymous, *J. Am. Pharm. Assoc., Pract. Pharm. Ed.*, **7**:158 (1946).

Anonymous, *J. Am. Pharm. Assoc., Pract. Pharm. Ed.*, **2**:290 (1941).

Anonymous, *J. Am. Pharm. Assoc., Pract. Pharm. Ed.*, **2**:467 (1941).

Anonymous, *J. Am. Pharm. Assoc., Pract. Pharm. Ed.*, **4**:31, 258, 335 (1943).

Anonymous, *J. Am. Pharm. Assoc., Pract. Pharm. Ed.*, **6**:293 (1945).

Jeffries, S. F., H. A. Nash, R. L. Harmon, D. C. Reynolds, and C. A. Bunde, *J. Am. Pharm. Assoc., Pract. Pharm. Ed.*, **13**:337 (1952).

Johnston, G. W., and C. O. Lee, *J. Am. Pharm. Assoc., Sci. Ed.*, **29**:236 (1940).

Johnston, G. W., and C. O. Lee, *J. Am. Pharm. Assoc., Sci. Ed.*, **32**:25 (1943).

Kettlitz, V., *Boll. Chim. Farm.*, Milano, **90**:2 (1951).

Klauder, J. B., E. R. Gross, and H. Brown, *Arch. Dermatol. Syphilol.*, **41**:331 (1940).

Kuever, R. A., and C. V. Burnside, *J. Am. Pharm. Assoc., Sci. Ed.*, **29**:373 (1940).

Kulchar, G. W., *Arch. Dermatol. Syphilol.*, **44**:43 (1941).

Kumer, L., *Dermat. Kosmetik*, Vienna (1949).

Kvorning, S. A., *Thesis*, Copenhagen (1949).

Landon, S., and L. C. Zopf, *J. Amer. Pharm. Assoc., Pract. Pharm. Ed.*, **4**:251 (1943).

LeRoux, M. H., *Bull. soc. franc. dermatol. syphilig.*, **47**:286 (1940).

Lesser, M. A., *Am. Profess. Pharmacist*, **19**:183 (1953).

Littlewood, S. D., *Pharm. J.*, **145**:85 (1940).

Lyman, R. A., *Pharmaceutical Compounding and Dispensing, 2nd Ed.*, Philadelphia, Lippincott (1955).

Mann, A., and F. Winter, *Die moderne Parfümerie*, Vienna (1932).

Martin, A.D., A. N. Marcus and C. O. Lee, *J. Am. Pharm. Assoc., Pract. Pharm. Ed.*, **14**:230 (1953).

Matthews, D.R., *Pharm. J.*, **148**:79 (1942).

Meyers, D.B., M. W. Nadkarin, and L. C. Zopf, *J. Am. Pharm. Assoc., Pract. Pharm. Ed.*, **11**:32 (1950).

Miller, J. L., M. H. Slatkin and B. A. Johnson, *Arch. Dermatol. Syphilol.*, **60**:106 (1949).

Miller, J. L., M. H. Slatkin, H. L. Wechsler, and B. A. Johnson., *Arch. Dermatol. Syphilol.*, **61**:648 (1950).

Mumford, P. B., *Brit. Med. J.*, **1**:266 (1939).

Mumford, P.B., *Brit. J. Dermatol. Syphilis*, **50**:540 (1938).

Mumford, P.B., and R. M. Mumford, *Brit. J. Dermatol. Syphilis*, **53**:45 (1941).

Newman, H., and O. H. Miller, *J. Am. Pharm. Assoc., Pract. Pharm. Ed.*, **15**:36 (1954).

Perrin, S. R., *Post Grad. Med.*, **8**:485 (1950).

Perrin, S. R., and A. Halpern, *J. Invest. Dermatol.*, **16**:7 (1951).

Pharmacopoeia Dancia (1948).

Pharmacopoeia Helvetica (1949).

Pharmacopoeia, Presbyterian Hosp., New York (1938).

Pillsbury, D. M., B. Shaefer, and A. C. Nichols, *J. Invest. Dermatol.*, **5**:371 (1942).

Polano, M. K., *Skin Therapeutics*, Houston, Elsevier Press (1952).
Polano, M. K., J. Bonsel, and B. J. VanderMeer, *Dermatologica*, **101**:69 (1950).
Powers, J. L., H. B. Leaske, and R. S. Warner, *J. Am. Pharm. Assoc., Pract. Pharm. Ed.*, **29**:14 (1940).
Jenkins, G. L., *Scoville's The Art of Compounding, 8th Ed.*, Philadelphia, Blakiston (1951).
Presslie, R., *Pharm. J.*, **157**:185 (1946).
Pribat, P., *Thesis*, Paris (1943).
Prinz, M. H. V., and L. P. Ereaus, *Can. Med. Assoc. J.*, **47**:344 (1942).
Quimby, S., and G. W. Fiero, *N. Y. State J. Med.*, **43**:157 (1943).
Rae, J., *Brit. J. Dermatol. Syphilis*, **65**:92 (1944).
Ray, L. F., and I. H. Blank, *Arch. Dermatol. Syphilol.*, **42**:285 (1940).
Redgrove, H. S., *Mfg. Chemist*, **14**:66 (1943).
Rigby, G., *Alchemist*, **16**:164 (1952).
Saute, R. E., and C. O. Lee, *J. Am. Pharm. Assoc., Pract. Pharm. Ed.*, **15**:39 (1954).
Scheineson, L. M., *Am. J. Ophth.*, **26**:171 (1943).
Schwartz, L., *Med. Clin. N. Amer.*, **26**:1195 (1942).
Soulsby, J., *Brit. J. Dermatol. Syphilis*, **52**:21, 25 (1940).
Soulsby, J., *Brit. J. Dermatol. Syphilis*, **61**:2-6 (1949).
Spalton, L. M., *Pharmaceutical Emulsions and Emulsifying Agents, 2nd Ed.*, New York, Chemical Publishing Co. (1953).
Strakosch, E. A., *J. Pharmacol. and Exp. Ther.*, **78**:65 (1943).
Sulzberger, M., *Current Med. Digest*, **20**:27 (1953).
Swallow, W., and T. D. Whittet, *Pharm. J.*, **147**:226 (1941).
Tyce, L. F., *Am. J. Pharm.*, **122**:131 (1950).
United States Pharmacopoeia 14th Rev. (1950).
Ward, J. B. and G. J. Sperandino, *J. Am. Pharm. Assoc., Prac. Pharm. Ed.*, **13**:98, 132 (1952).
Whittet, T. D., *Pharm. J.*, **150**:139 (1943).
Wood, W. C., *Pharm. J.*, **142**:327 (1939).
Yalcindag, O. N., *Am. J. Pharm.*, **124**:386 (1952).
Zopf, L. C., *J. Am. Pharm. Assoc., Prac. Pharm. Ed.*, **6**:365 (1945).

INDEX

A

Absobase, 115
Absorption Base, 15
Absorptive Bases, 15
Actibase, 140
Adalotion, 85
Adbase, 56
Agralotion, 97
Agualotion, 70
Albabase, 56
Aliphatic Alcohols, 13
Allolotion, 105
Alpabase, 49
Altabase, 44
Altibase, 47
Amibase, 45
Amine Derivatives, 16
Ammonium Salts, Quaternary, 13
Anabase, 139
Anhydrous Bases, 15, 16
Anhydrous Washable Oil-in-Water Unguent Bases 130
Anhydrous Water-in-Oil Nonwashable Unguent Bases, 136
Anionic Surface-Active Agents, 13
Antibiotics, 16, 18
Applilotion, 124
Aqueous Phase, 12, 13
Armabase, 39
Atherbase, 21
Autobase, 25

B

Basibase, 24
Beebase, 114
Beeswax, 17
Bemabase, 27
Benzalkonium Chloride, 13
Berabase, 108
Besslotion, 81
Betabase, 29
Bevabase, 48
Bibliography, 141
Bodibase, 113
Body of Anhydrous Bases, 15
Bonabase, 137
Bornibase, 27
Breaking of the Emulsion, 13
Briabase, 31

Buffabase, 19

C

Calmlotion, 101
Carbowaxes, 14, 15
Carrier. See Vehicle.
Cationic Surface Active Agents, 13
Cellulose Derivatives, 16
Centralotion, 95
Cetilotion, 78
Cetobase, 51
Cetyl Alcohol, 14, 17
Charilotion, 103
Cherilotion, 123
Cholebase, 116
Cholesterol, 14, 17
Claralotion, 105
Clerabase, 112
Clymalotion, 78
Compatibility of Drugs, 18
Complotion, 94
Creamlotion, 92
Credobase, 139
Crembase, 42

D

Dactobase, 109
Dalbase, 110
Dalylotion, 99
Darlotion, 98
Deaclotion, 79
Debubase, 35
Dekabase, 64
Deltalotion, 125
Deltilotion, 95
Delvilotion, 90
Demibase, 59
Depabase, 115
Derabase, 36
Dermal Penetration, 14, 15
Desabase, 53
Desorbase, 134
Detrilotion, 104
Diabase, 111
Dilubase, 57
Diplobase, 26
Dispersing Agent, 16
Doebase, 58
Dolbase, 55
Donabase, 21
Drug Inactivation, 17
Drug Stability, 18
Dual Action of Surface-Active Agents, 14
Duralotion, 68
Dynabase, 25

E

Edelbase, 132
Edylotion, 68
Effbase, 52
Effective Therapy, 16
Elbalotion, 102
Elilotion, 77
Elmbase, 39
Emolibase, 24
Emollients, 15
Emulsibase, 53
Emulsifying Agent, Choice of, 13
Emulsion, Breaking of, 13
Emulsion Stability, 16
Emulsions, Oil-in-Water 13
Emulsions, Water-in-Oil 13
Entrobase, 110
Equabase, 42
Equilibrium between Water

Loss and Water Gain, 15
Ergolotion, 76
Erthalotion, 85
Estabase, 113
Ethibase, 44
Eurobase, 62
Everbase, 34
Exobase, 19
External Phase, 13

F

Fairbase, 131
Fatty Acid Glyceryl Esters, 13, 14
Fatty Acids, Sorbitol Compounds of, 13
Fatty Acids, Sorbitol Esters of, 14
Fatty Alcohols, 14, 16
Feldlotion, 74
Finlotion, 66
Floralotion, 99
Fortabase, 136

G

Gardobase, 114
Geobase, 59
Genalotion, 81
Gentilotion, 70
Glycerin, 15, 17
Glycerin Substitute, 14
Glyceryl Esters, 16
Glyceryl Esters of Fatty Acids, 13, 14
Glyceryl Monostearate, 13, 17
Glycol Derivatives, 16
Granbase, 37
Gretabase, 135

H

H Base, 35
Hastibase, 45
Heilbase, 46
Hetribase, 28
Homogenization, 16
Hospilotion, 128
Humabase, 28
Humectant, 14, 15
Hydrophilic, 12, 14
Hylobase, 30

I

Inactivation of Drugs, 17
Incompatibility, 18
Ingredients of Lotions, Common, 17
Ingredients of Unguent Bases, Common, 17
Internal Phase, 13
Intobase, 117
Introduction, 11
Ionic Charge, 12
Irabase, 57
Ivabase, 53
Ivilotion, 67

J

Jefbase, 46
Jeribase, 60
Jordalotion, 92

K

Kebrabase, 41
Kenilotion, 125
Kestilotion, 83
Ketabase, 130
Keybase, 43

Kombalotion, 96

L

Lanolin, 15, 17
Lanolin Derivatives, 16
Largobase, 33
Latabase, 118
Laurabase, 41
Laurolotion, 85
Librabase, 38
Lipophilic, 12, 14
Lipophilic Portion, 13
Liqualotion, 127
Liquid Content of Lotions, 12
Liquid Content of Unguent Bases, 12
Liquid Petrolatum, 17
Lochlotion, 100
Lodolotion, 86
Loftlotion, 67
Logabase, 26
Longlotion, 84

M

Majorlotion, 71
Marmalotion, 75
Maylotion, 87
Melobase, 54
Melolotion, 65
Metallic Salts, 16
Methyl Cellulose, 17
Methyl Paraaminobenzoate, 15
Methyl Paraben, 17
Miralotion, 126
Mistlotion, 72
Modibase, 20
Mold Growth, 15
Monalotion, 74
Monbase, 63

N

Natalotion, 69
Natural Gums, 16
Naxilotion, 90
Neetlotion, 77
Neutralizing the Therapeutic Action, 17
Nirolotion, 124
Nonionic Emulsifiers, 14
Nonionic Surface-Active Agents, 13, 14
Nonwashable Bases, 16
Nonwashable Water-in-Oil Anhydrous Unguent Bases, 136
Nonwashable Water-in-Oil Lotions, 120
Nonwashable Water-in-Oil Unguent Bases, 108
Normabase, 51
Normalotion, 96
Notobase, 29
Novalotion, 121
Nubase, 63
Nybase, 47

O

Oborlotion, 82
Oil Phase, 12
Oil-in-Water, Definition of the Term, 13
Oil-in-Water Emulsions, 13, 14, 15, 16
Oil-in-Water Washable Anhydrous Unguent Bases, 130
Oil-in-Water Washable Lotions, 65
Oil-in-Water Washable Unguent Bases, 19

Oils, 16
Oil-Soluble Ingredients, 17
Oil-Soluble Surface-Active Agents, 16
Oily Emollient, 14
Oleaginous Substances, 13, 14
Olilotion, 127
Ontobase, 117
Operalotion, 127
Ornabase, 37
Ortholotion, 80
Oslerbase, 32
Ovabase, 118

P

Padbase, 50
Parabens, 15
Paralotion, 71
Parbase, 138
Parmabase, 37
Particle Size, 16
Partlotion, 89
Pelulotion, 80
Penetration into the Skin, 15
Perlbase, 23
Permibase, 30
Perrilotion, 68
Petrolatum, 16, 17
Petrolotion, 96
Pettibase, 43
Pharmlotion, 87
Pharmolotion, 123
Physibase, 137
Physician, Role of, 15
Plibase, 132
Polotion, 84
Polyethylene Glycol Derivatives, 14
Polyethylene Glycols, 15, 17
Portlotion, 77
Portolotion, 93
Practolotion, 94
Pregobase, 40
Prenalotion, 106
Propabase, 58
Properties of Lotions, 11
Properties of Unguent Bases 11
Propyl Paraaminobenzoate, 15
Propyl Paraben, 17
Propylene Glycol, 17
Protective Agents, 15
Protolotion, 104
Provalotion, 88
Provolotion, 72
Pyalotion, 102

Q

Qualibase, 137
Quaternary Ammonium Salts, 13

R

Regulotion, 107
Release of Drugs, 18
Renobase, 33
Retobase, 133
Retrobase, 31
Reylotion, 106
Rimbase, 25
Rinobase, 116
Romabase, 31
Rosalotion, 72
Rowbase, 54

S

Sadlotion, 122

Salicylic Acid, 16
Saltilotion, 120
Sanabase, 52
Sarlotion, 93
Sedlotion, 73
Seebase, 48
Segualotion, 92
Selflotion, 82
Semabase, 134
Septalotion, 79
Serenbase, 131
Serralotion, 89
Sharlotion, 99
Sidrolotion, 76
Silkbase, 112
Simolotion, 126
Sindlotion, 88
Sintrabase, 36
Sirbase, 62
Situbase, 140
Skin, Penetration into, 15
Soaps, 13, 16
Sodium Alkly Sulfonate, 12
Sodium Lauryl Sulfate, 13
Sofbase, 20
Solalotion, 66
Sorbitan Laurate, 14
Sorbitan Monooleate, 13
Sorbitan Oleate, 14
Sorbitan Stearate, 14
Sorbitol, 14, 17
Sorbitol Compounds of Fatty Acids, 13
Sorbitol Esters of Fatty Acids, 14
Sorbitol Fatty Acid Esters, 16
Spans, 14
Sparobase, 23
Specilotion, 103
Spermaceti, 17
Sponbase, 109
Sprilotion, 75
Spyrolotion, 103
Stability of Drugs, 18
Stability of Emulsion, 16
Stearic Acid, 17
Stearyl Alcohol, 14, 17
Stefbase, 49
Stemlotion, 121
Sterabase, 50
Studabase, 139
Sulfated Fatty Acid Derivatives, 16
Sulfur, 16
Sunbase, 49
Suprabase, 34
Surface-Active Agents, 12, 13
Surface-Active Agents, Common, 16
Surface-Active Agents, Dual Action of, 14
Surfalotion, 69

T

Tactilotion, 98
Tatalotion, 91
Tectilotion, 73
Templotion, 65
Thanlotion, 83
Theralotion, 81
Therapeutic Agents, Water-Sensitive, 16
Tonabase, 60
Toplotion, 91
Torobase, 22
Totabase, 138
Tramlotion, 84
Transibase, 22

Trimlotion, 107
Trubase, 61
Trulotion, 97
Tuabase, 59
Tweens, 14
Type of Emulsions, 13
Tyrobase, 111

U

Unguabase, 133

V

Varibase, 40
Vehicle, 15
Verdibase, 108
Vernalotion, 122
Viscosity of Anhydrous Bases, 15
Vitrabase, 136
Vivalotion, 101

W

Waralotion, 87
Washability, 14, 15
Washable Anhydrous Oil-in-Water Unguent Bases 130
Washable Oil-in-Water Lotions, 65
Washable Oil-in-Water Unguent Bases, 19
Water, 17
Water Content, 15
Water Gain, 15
Water Loss, 15
Water-Dispersible Agents, 12
Water-in-Oil, Definition of the Term, 13
Water-in-Oil Emulsions, 13, 14, 16
Water-in-Oil Lotions, Nonwashable, 120
Water-in-Oil Nonwashable Anhydrous Unguent Bases, 136
Water-in-Oil Nonwashable Unguent Bases, 108
Water-in-Oil Unguent Bases, 14
Water-Sensitive Therapeutic Agents, 16
Water-Soluble Agents, 12
Water-Soluble Ingredients, 17
Water-Soluble Surface-Active Agents, 16
Wax Substitutes, 15
Welbase, 61
Well-Balanced Formula, 15
Whitbase, 55
Willotion, 99
Winbase, 63
Withlotion, 128
Wunbase, 130

Z

Zonabase, 38
Zonalotion, 120

www.ingramcontent.com/pod-product-compliance
Lightning Source LLC
LaVergne TN
LVHW022052200926
848481LV00003B/878